I dedicate this book to my son Zach who bears with me in my "nature girl" and "Hippie" ways and lifestyle and supports me in all I do. Thanks son I love you very much!

Introduction

Hello, my name is Veronica I am a soap maker, artist, photographer, book writer, jewelry maker, and I am working on becoming an aroma therapist. I am an all around crafty gal that lives to create and make beautiful things. I have always been interested in natural things. I do my best to go green and natural whenever I can and I am working on making it a way of life. I own a soap making business (The Cupertino Soap Company) and 7 years ago got certified as a Green Business in the State of California which was a really big deal for me. So I strive to be more earth friendly and continue to work on a green lifestyle. I am fortunate to have a wonderful herb garden and vegetable garden from which I can get lots of natural botanicals that I can use to make natural products.

I am always working on a new recipe for natural body products, or a safer way to clean my house. I really don't like using a lot of chemicals it's not good for the planet or our bodies. I have been experimenting with a lot of ways to be more green, hence this book. I wanted to share it with other people.

Most of the recipes you find in this book can be made with simple ingredients and things you can find in your kitchen and home. I have listed some resources at the end of this book for the other ingredients you may not have at home. All of these recipes are easy to follow and don't require a lot of special equipment. I have made a list of items for you that would be handy to have and help you make your homemade products.

Each recipe has an ingredient list, clear easy directions, how to use it and I explain the benefits of the ingredients so that you can understand what they do and how they will be good for your body or your home. I have done a lot of research over the years on essential oils, natural cleaning agents, herbs and other natural ingredients that benefit a green lifestyle. I hope you enjoy the book!

Contents

Beauty Products ....page 5

Household Cleaning Products...........page 39

Health Products ....page 61

Easy Aromatherapy............................page 78

Resources...page 87

Index..page 88

A list of some of the things to have on hand

Various sizes of glass mason jars with plastic lids
Small food processor or coffee grinder
Essential Oils such as: Lavender, Chamomile, Rosemary, Eucalyptus, Orange, Peppermint.
Dried Herbs and flowers such as: Lavender, Chamomile, Calendula, Roses
Oils to have: Coconut oil, Olive oil, Almond Oil
Double Boiler
White and Apple Cider Vinegar
Bees Wax
Witch Hazel
Rubbing Alcohol
Spray Bottles of various sizes
Castile Soap
Borax
Peroxide
Aloe Vera
Shower Cap
Silicon molds (like for cupcakes or ice cubes)
Inexpensive Vodka
Small mixing bowls
Measuring Spoons
Measuring Cups
A small food scale

Caution – Never use essential oils in the eyes or mucus membranes. Do not take them internally without the supervision of a professional medical practitioner. Be sure not to use undiluted essential oil on the skin, properly dilute the oil with carrier oil such as olive, almond oil, etc. I make no claims to be a health care professional. This information is for educational purposes only and this information has not been evaluated by the FDA. This information is not intended to diagnose, treat, cure or prevent any disease.

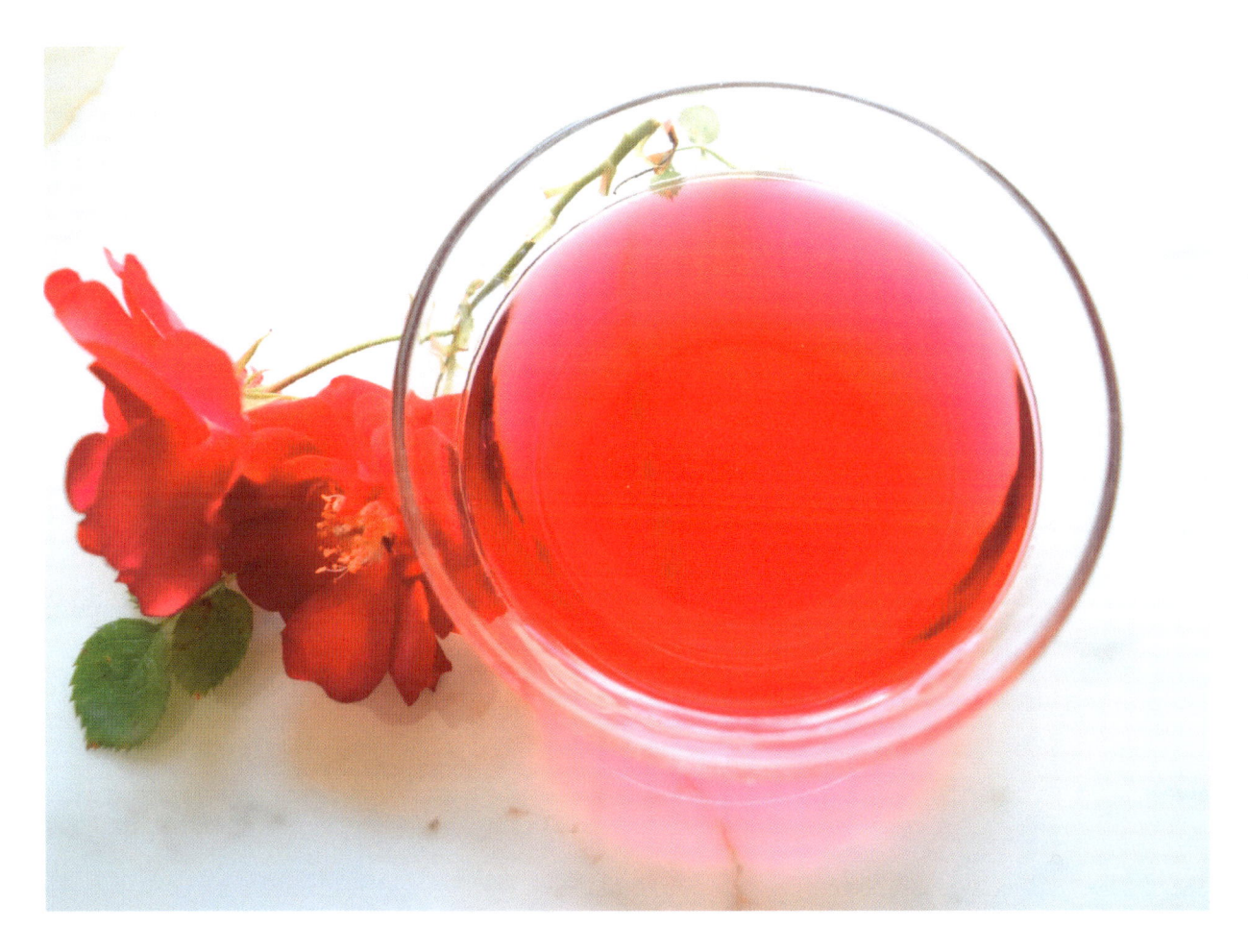

Beauty Products

You don't need chemicals in your beauty routine. There is so much you can make on your own with wonderful all natural ingredients you probably already have right in your kitchen. You can turn ordinary coconut oil and sugar into a wonderful body scrub, or use olive oil for an organic hair conditioner. You can even make a dry shampoo with corn starch. This section will show you how to do just that. Each recipe will list all the ingredients you need and step by step directions. Be sure to check the list of things that are handy to have before you start making your own lovely beauty treatments.

Rose Infused Witch Hazel

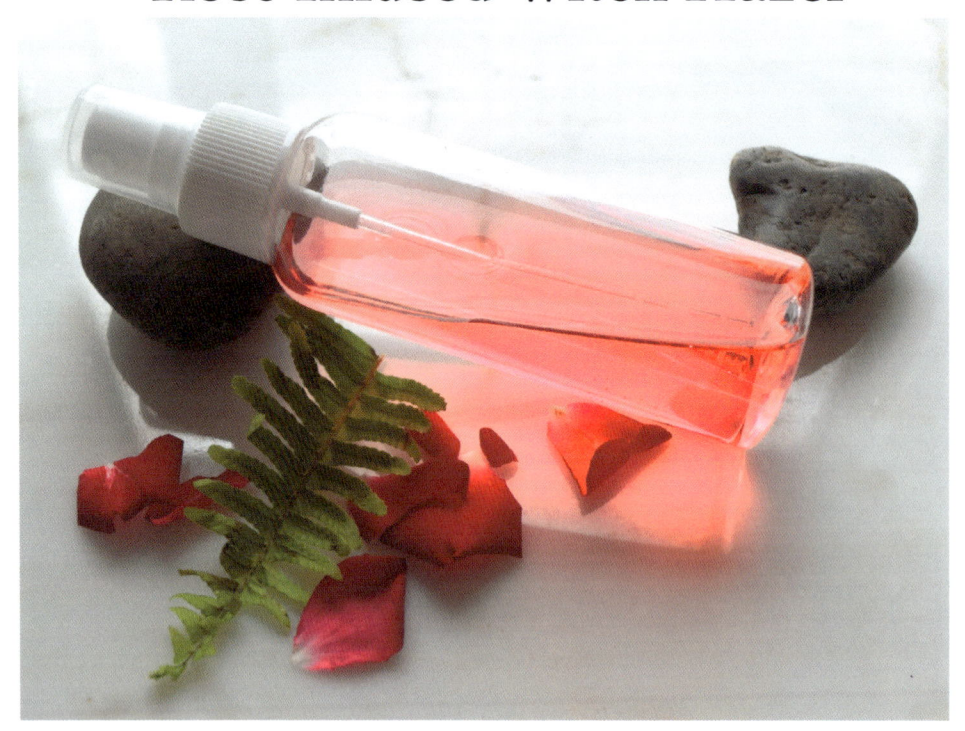

Ingredients:

fresh rose petals (only use petals from roses without pesticides or chemicals*)
witch hazel
1 quart mason jar with a plastic lid

Directions:

Gather fresh rose petals from your bushes. Wash them thoroughly and dry them. Fill the jar all the way to the top with the petals but don't pack the petals too tightly. Pour the witch hazel over the petals until the jar is full. Let sit in a cool dark place for several days until the mixture turns a pinkish/red color then strain out the petals and store in a Mason jar.

How to Use: Witch hazel is an astringent and antiseptic, so it is helpful for spot controlling acne or used as an overall facial toner.

Benefits:

If you have rose bushes you have a gold mine in your garden! Roses are well known for their lovely fragrance and their rose hips that are full of vitamin C. The flowers have skin refreshing properties. The antioxidants in roses protect the cells in the skin against damage. Rose also has anti-inflammatory properties, which means it can be put on the skin to soothe irritation. Roses have antiseptic and antibacterial properties; it can help wounds heal faster by keeping them clean and fighting infections. Witch hazel is a plant that is native to North America, the bark and leaves are used to make a skin healing astringent.

*If you don't have a rose bush you can buy dried rose petals and use them.

Rose Water

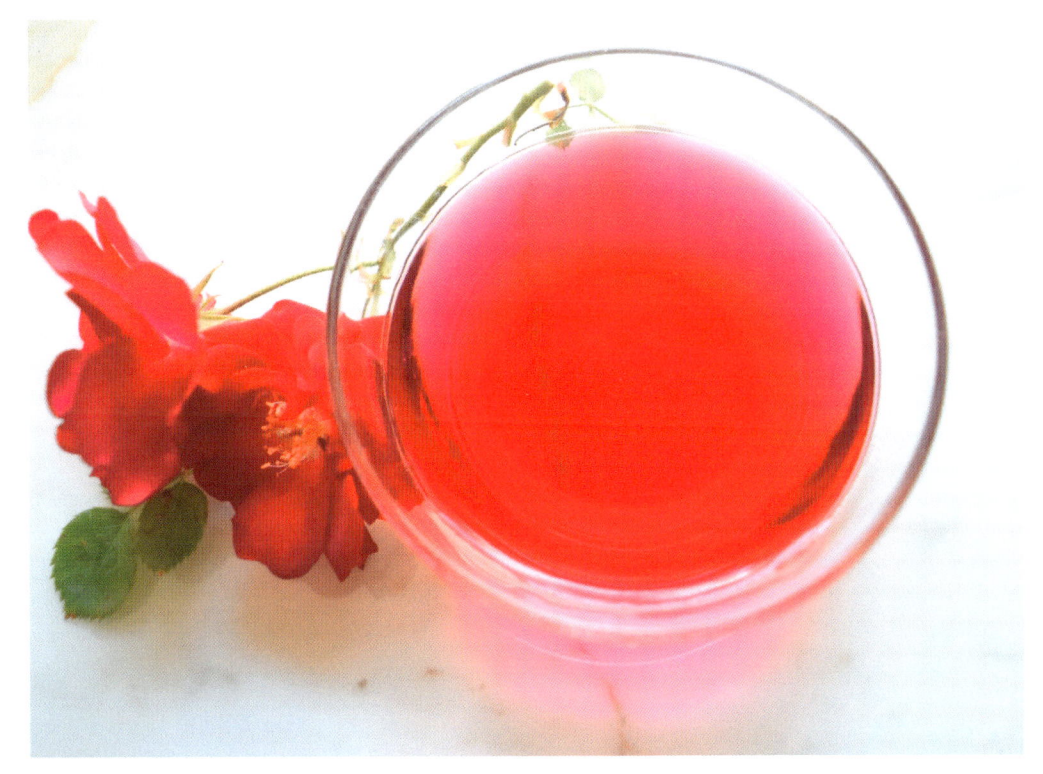

Ingredients:

Fresh rose petals (only use petals from roses without pesticides or chemicals*)
glass jar to store your rosewater in
distilled water

Directions:

Add petals to a large pot and top with enough distilled water to just cover the rose petals. Let simmer for 20-30 minutes or until petals have lost their color and are a pale pink. Strain the mixture to separate the petals from the water. Discard petals and place water in a glass jar to store.

How to use:

You can use for cooking, baking or as a face toner. Store in the refrigerator in an airtight container.

*If you don't have a rose bush you can buy dried rose petals and use them.

Benefits:

The antioxidants in rose water protect the cells in the skin against damage. Rose water also has anti-inflammatory properties, which means it can be put on the skin to soothe irritation. Rose water has antiseptic and antibacterial properties; it can help wounds heal faster by keeping them clean and fighting infections. Cooking with rose water adds a light floral taste to your food.

Calendula and Rose Hip Facial Serum

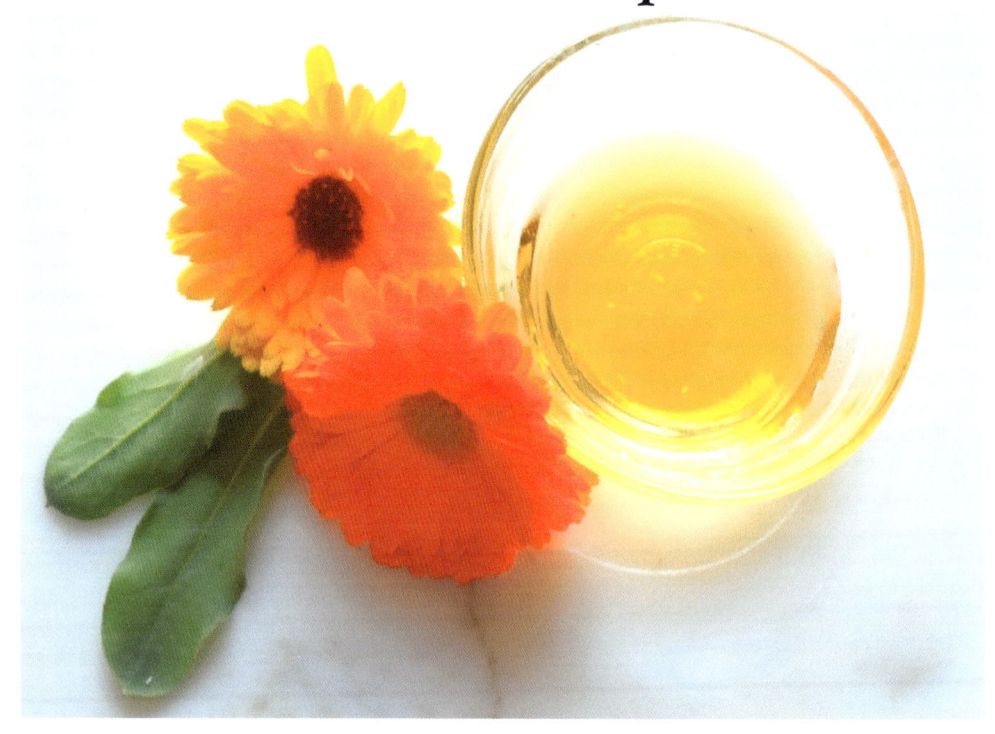

Ingredients:

1 oz rose hip seed oil
1 oz Calendula infused grape seed oil *
1 oz jojoba oil
10 drops carrot seed essential oil
5 drops chamomile essential oil
10 drops of vitamin E oil
small bottle to store your serum in

Directions: In a small bowl add all the ingredients and mix until all is combined. Pour into a small bottle. Store in a cool dark place.

*Calendula infused oil Directions:

Fill a glass jar 2/3 of the way full with dried Calendula flowers. Pour oil into the jar, making sure to cover the flowers by at least one inch with oil so they will have space to expand. Stir well and cap the jar tightly. Place the jar in a warm, sunny windowsill and shake once or more daily. After 4 to 6 weeks, strain the herbs out using cheesecloth. Pour the infused oil into a glass bottle and store in a cool, dark place.

How to use: Apply a small amount morning and night to your face.

Benefits: Rose hips seed oil is very high in vitamin C which is considered to be beneficial to skin cell regeneration. Grape seed oil is high in vitamins, minerals and polyunsaturated fatty acids. It is believed to preserve the natural moisture in aging skin. Carrot seed oil is thought to have the ability to regenerate mature skin cells and may help promote tone and elasticity to skin. Carrot seed oil has potent antioxidant properties; it has vitamin A and minerals. Calendula has anti-fungal, anti-inflammatory and antibacterial properties that could help heal wounds, and sooth dry skin.

Anti-Aging Face Cream

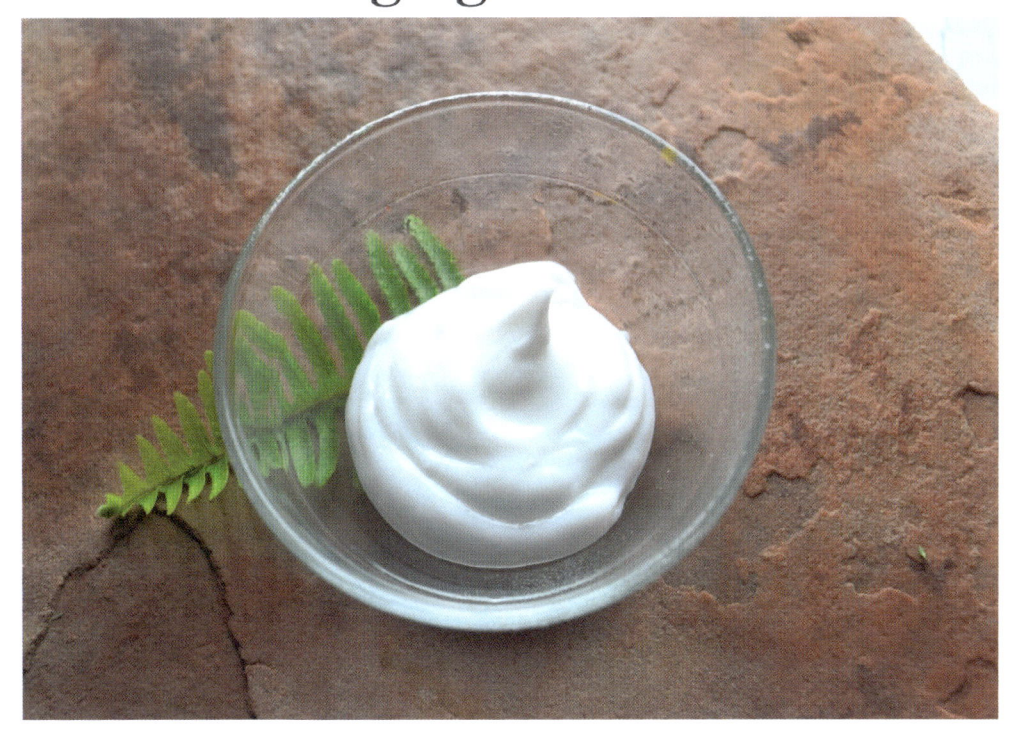

Ingredients:

1/4 cup almond oil
2 tablespoons coconut oil
1 tablespoon of grated beeswax
or beeswax pellets
1/2 teaspoon vitamin E oil
5 drops of geranium essential oil

1 tablespoon Shea butter
10 drops of carrot seed oil
small glass jar to store it in

Directions: Place all ingredients in a double boiler. Melt the oils, butters and wax on medium low. Stir occasionally. Once the mixture has melted and all is evenly combined, pour it into a small glass jar. Let it sit at room temperature until the cream cools, then cover. Store in a cool place.

How to use: Apply morning and night after washing your face.

Benefits: Geranium essential oil is a good skin toner. The scent is soothing, mood lifting and balancing. It can help with eczema. Carrots aren't just good for your eyes; they are also good for your skin. Carrot seed oil is thought to have the ability to regenerate mature skin cells and may help promote tone and elasticity to skin. Carrot seed oil has potent antioxidant properties. It has vitamin A and minerals. Carrot seed oil can help sooth inflamed or sensitive skin. Shea butter also has anti-inflammatory and healing properties. Using Shea butter on your body, especially your face, can condition, tone, and soothe your skin. Coconut oil may be linked to some potential benefits for skin including; reducing inflammation, keeping skin moisturized and helping heal wounds. The medium-chain fatty acids found in coconut oil also possess antimicrobial properties that can help treat acne and protect the skin from harmful bacteria.

Green Tea Toner

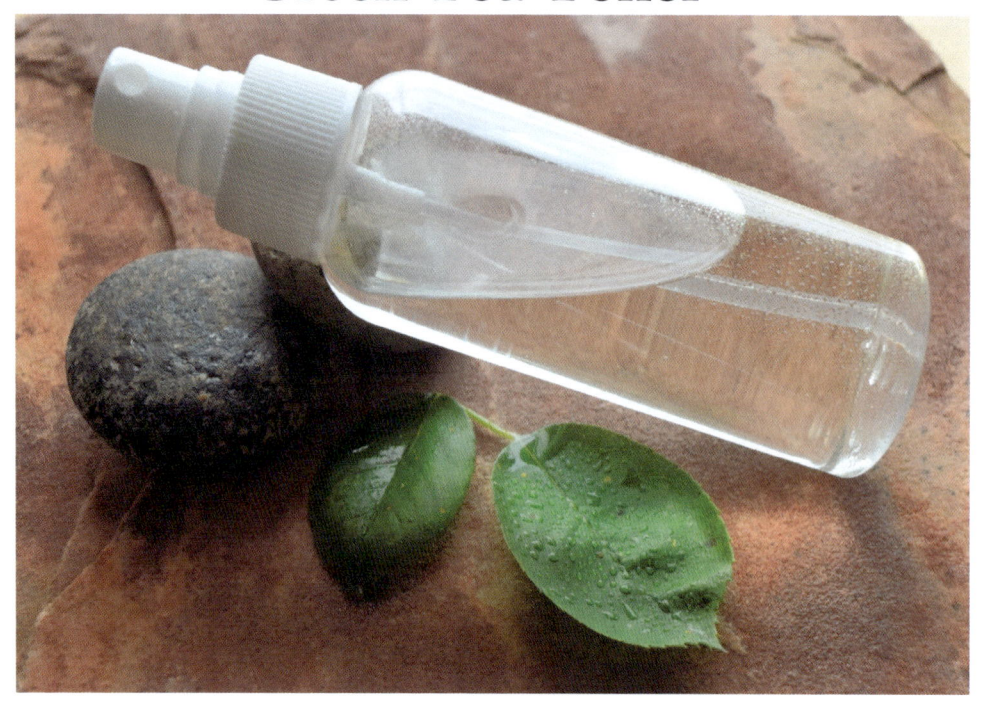

Ingredients:

1/4 cup of fresh brewed organic green tea
1 tablespoon organic apple cider vinegar
5 drops frankincense essential oil
1 drops lemon grass essential oil
5 drops lavender essential oil
2 ounce bottle

Directions:

Mix all ingredients in the spray bottle and shake well.

How to use:

Gently apply with a cotton ball and avoid eyes. Use this toner up within 1-2 weeks.

Benefits:

Green tea contains a powerful antioxidant called EGCG that fights DNA damage from UV rays to prevent skin cancer. That means it's also a potent anti-aging ingredient that combats signs of aging when ingested or applied topically. Frankincense will soothe and reduce inflammation and the boswellic acids it contains are capable of killing bacteria associated with acne. Lemon grass is an antibacterial, anti-fungal and anti-inflammatory. Lavender has been used since ancient times to purify and cleanse. The essential oil has healing properties for the skin. Lavender essential oil has natural antibacterial and antidepressant properties.

Oat Honey Facial Mask

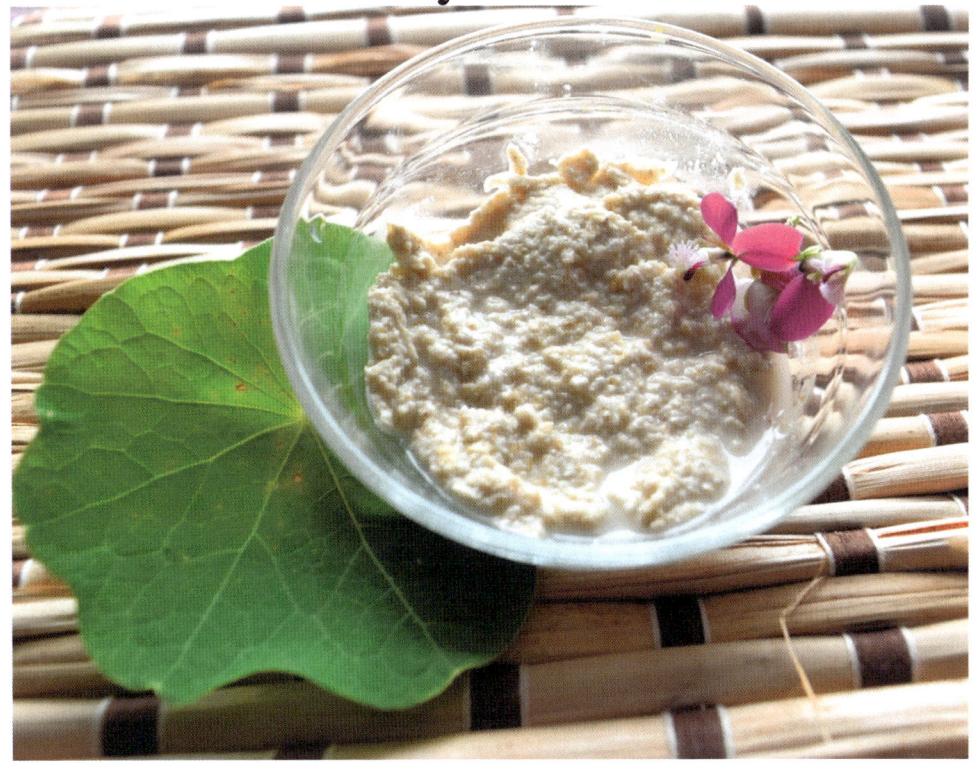

Ingredients:

1/4 cup of ground oatmeal
1 1/2 tablespoons of honey
1–2 teaspoon of water

Directions:

Grind oatmeal in a clean coffee grinder, blender or mini food processor. Mix oatmeal with honey and add a little bit of water to make a paste.

To use: Gently spread on face, let sit for 5-10 minutes wipe off with a damp cloth then rinse your face.

Benefits:

The oatmeal will exfoliate the skin and the honey has natural antibacterial properties. When oatmeal is hydrated it naturally moisturizes and creates a protective barrier on the skin. It also acts as a natural pore cleanser, and is soothing to sensitive skin. Honey has antibacterial and antiseptic properties, so it gets rid of dirt and bacteria, which is perfect for both preventing and treating acne. It's full of antioxidants and boosts collagen production. It's extremely moisturizing and hydrates even the driest of skin. Honey is naturally soothing and has healing properties. It works as a clarifying agent because it naturally opens up pores, making them easier to unclog.

Yogurt Mint Cucumber Facial Mask

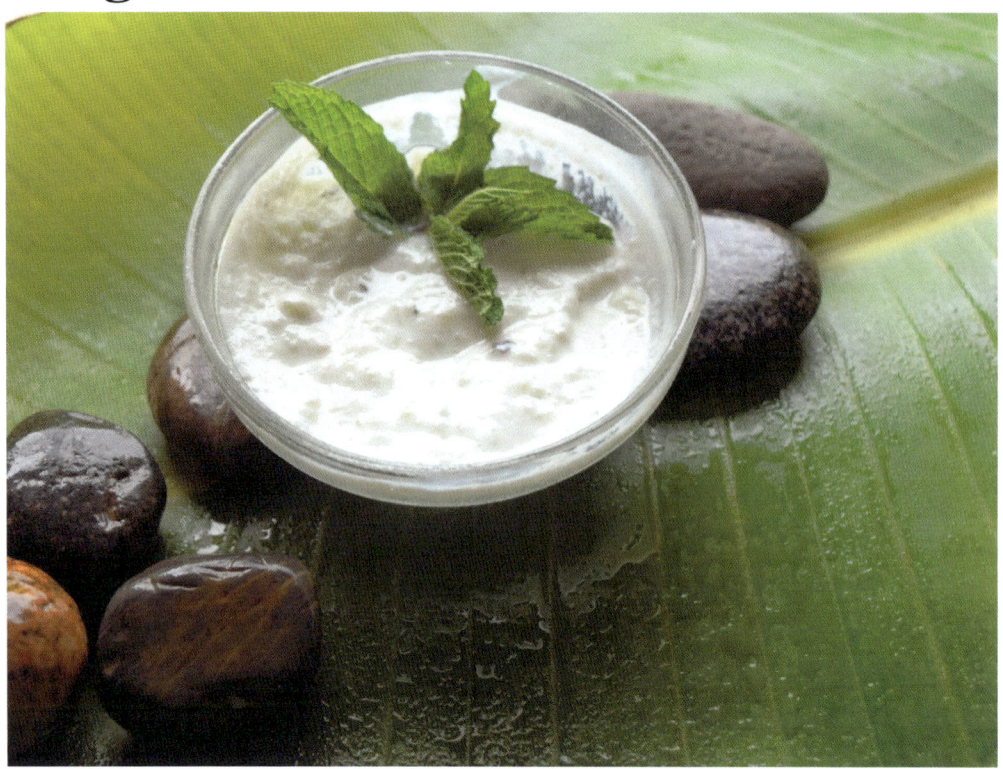

Ingredients:

2 tablespoons fresh mint leaves, rinsed, dried, and chopped
1/2 cup plain yogurt
2 tablespoons white Kaolin clay
4 slices of cucumber

Directions:

Add all of the ingredients to a small food processor or small drink blender and blend well until all ingredients are incorporated. Remove the mixture and transfer it to a clean container. Refrigerate the mixture for up to three days, and then discard it.

To use:

Simply add a small amount to cover your face and let sit for 15 minutes then rinse off.

Benefits:

The lactic acid in yogurt gently exfoliates the skin while the Kaolin clay draws out toxins and dirt that can clog pores and dull your complexion. Fresh mint gives this mask a cool, invigorating aroma that will leave you feeling wonderfully refreshed.

Deep Cleansing Facial Mud Mask

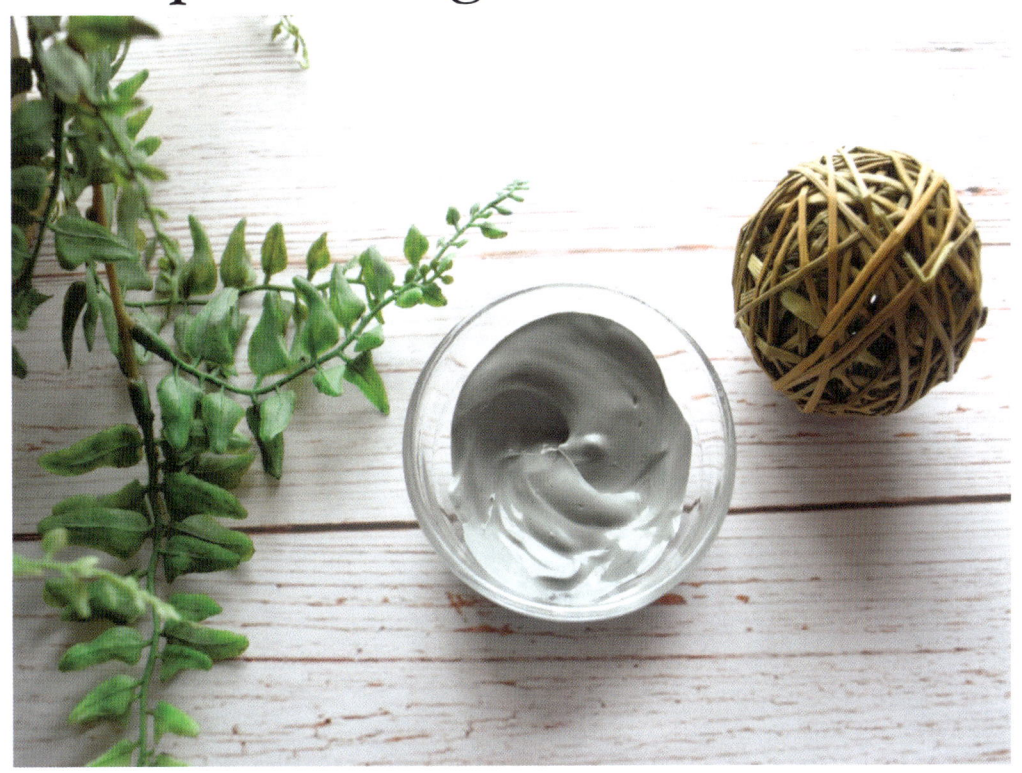

Ingredients:

1 tablespoon Dead Sea mud powder
1 1/2 teaspoons olive oil
5 drops spearmint essential oil
2 drops tea tree essential oil
2 slices of cucumber

Directions:

In a small mixing bowl, combine the Dead Sea mud powder and olive oil. Mix well to combine, than add the essential oils and mix again.

How to use:

This mask is best used fresh. Apply it liberally to moistened skin, avoiding your eyes, and lips. Discard the leftover. Cover your eyes with slices of fresh cucumber, and then relax for 10-15 minutes. Rinse the mask away, and follow with your favorite toner and moisturizer.

Benefits:

Dead Sea mud reduces skin impurities. Mud masks can work to remove impurities and dead skin on your body and face. An added benefit of Dead Sea mud is that the salt and magnesium in it can improve your skin's functionality by making it a better barrier and more elastic. Tea tree essential oil is known for its antibacterial properties.

Clay Face Mask

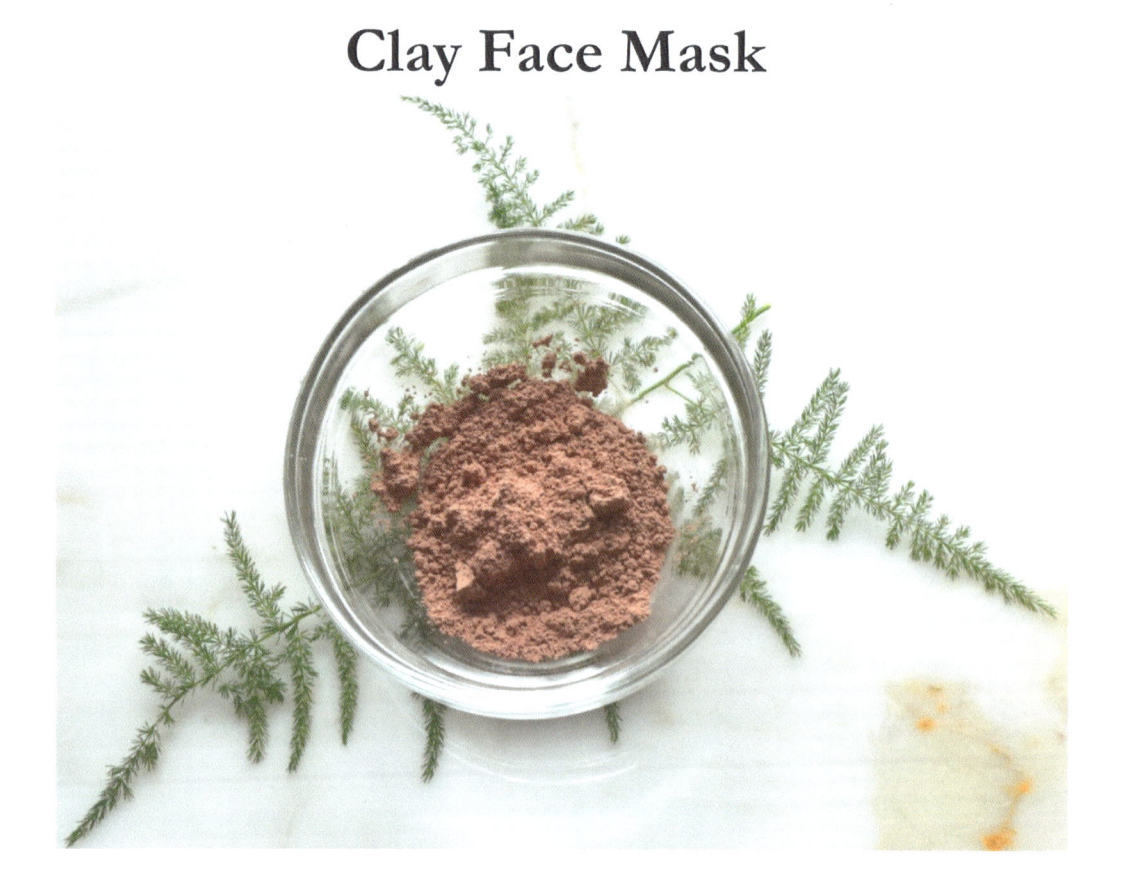

Ingredients:

2 teaspoons French green clay (or substitute kaolin or rose clay for sensitive/dry skin)
4-5 teaspoons aloe vera gel
1 teaspoon of honey

Directions:

In a small bowl mix the clay and the aloe vera gel, then add the honey.

How to use:

Put a thin layer on your face using your fingers. Let set for 15 minutes then rinse off with warm water.

Benefits:

Clay detoxifies and purifies the skin, it unclogs and shrinks pores and improves skin tone. Honey has antibacterial and anti-septic properties, so it gets rid of dirt and bacteria, perfect for both preventing and treating acne. It's full of antioxidants and boosts collagen production. It's extremely moisturizing and hydrates even the driest of skin. Honey is naturally soothing and has healing properties. It works as a clarifying agent because it naturally opens up pores, making them easier to unclog. Aloe vera contains antioxidants, enzymes, vitamins A and C, and it is highly anti-inflammatory. It can help treat burns, acne and dry skin.

Facial Clay Mask

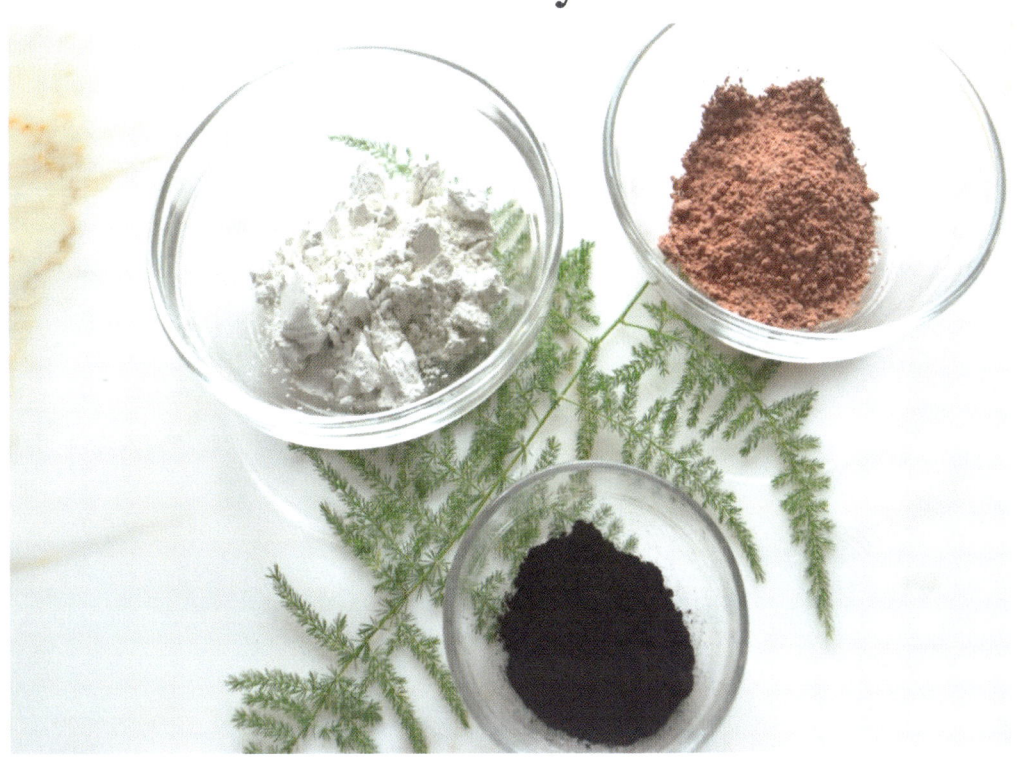

Ingredients:

small jar about 4 ounces
4 tablespoons of honey
1/4 cup of Kaolin Pink French or Bentonite clay
10 drops of lavender or chamomile essential oil

Directions: In a small bowl mix the clay and honey then add the essential oil. Store in a small glass jar with a lid in the refrigerator.

How to use:

Put a thin layer on your face using your fingers. Let set for 15 minutes then rinse off with warm water.

Benefits:

Clay detoxifies and purifies the skin, it unclogs and shrinks pores and improves skin tone. Honey has antibacterial and anti-septic properties, so it gets rid of dirt and bacteria, perfect for both preventing and treating acne. It's full of antioxidants and boosts collagen production. Honey is extremely moisturizing and hydrates even the driest of skin. It is naturally soothing and has healing properties. It works as a clarifying agent because it naturally opens up pores, making them easier to unclog. Lavender essential oil has wonderful healing properties for the skin; it helps relieve itchy skin and acne. Chamomile helps fade spots, eliminate acne scars and fight breakouts, due to its anti-inflammatory and antiseptic properties. Chamomile is a powerhouse of antioxidants and protects the skin from free-radical damage.

Cooling Cucumber Facial Mask

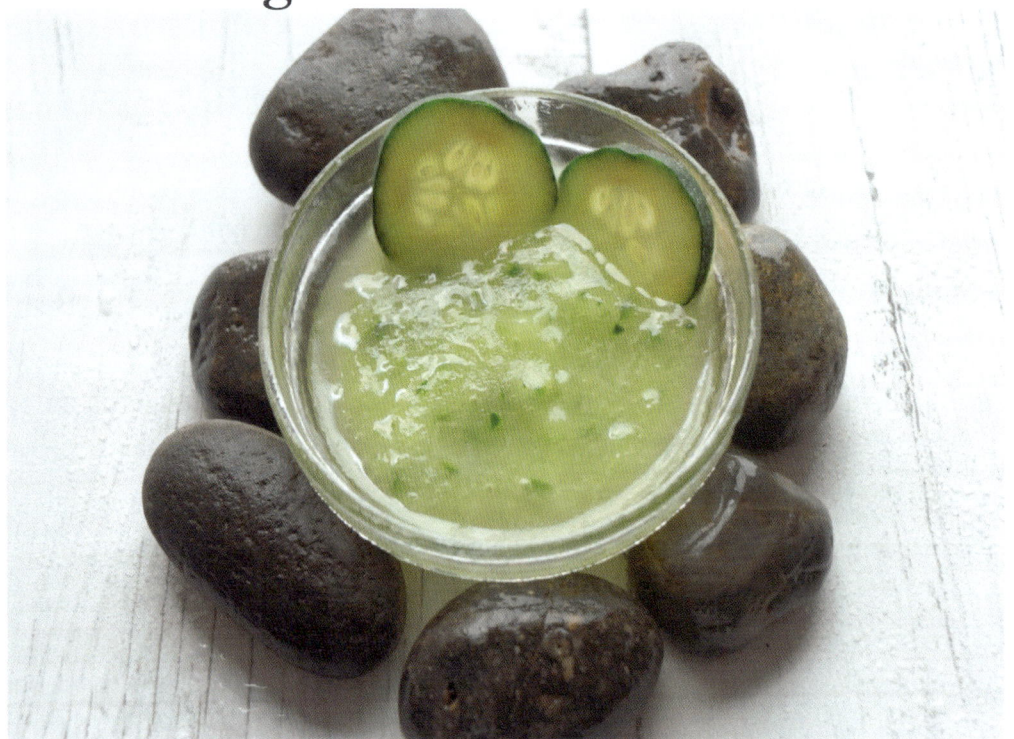

Ingredients:

1/4 of a cucumber
2 tablespoons coconut oil
1/4 cup aloe vera gel
8 drops of carrot seed essential oil

Directions:

Blend all ingredients together in a small food processor or drink blender until it forms a smooth cream. Store in an air tight container in the refrigerator for one week.

How to use:

Apply to the face and let set for 15 minutes then rinse.

Benefits:

Aloe vera contains antioxidants, enzymes, vitamins A and C, and it is highly anti-inflammatory. It can help treat burns, acne and dry skin. Coconut oil may be linked to some potential benefits for skin, including reducing inflammation, keeping skin moisturized and helping heal wounds. The medium-chain fatty acids found in coconut oil also possess antimicrobial properties that can help treat acne and protect the skin from harmful bacteria. Carrot seed oil is thought to have the ability to regenerate mature skin cells and may help promote tone and elasticity to skin. Carrot seed oil has potent antioxidant properties; it has vitamin A and minerals. Cucumber reduces puffiness and cools the skin.

Oatmeal and Clay Facial Scrub

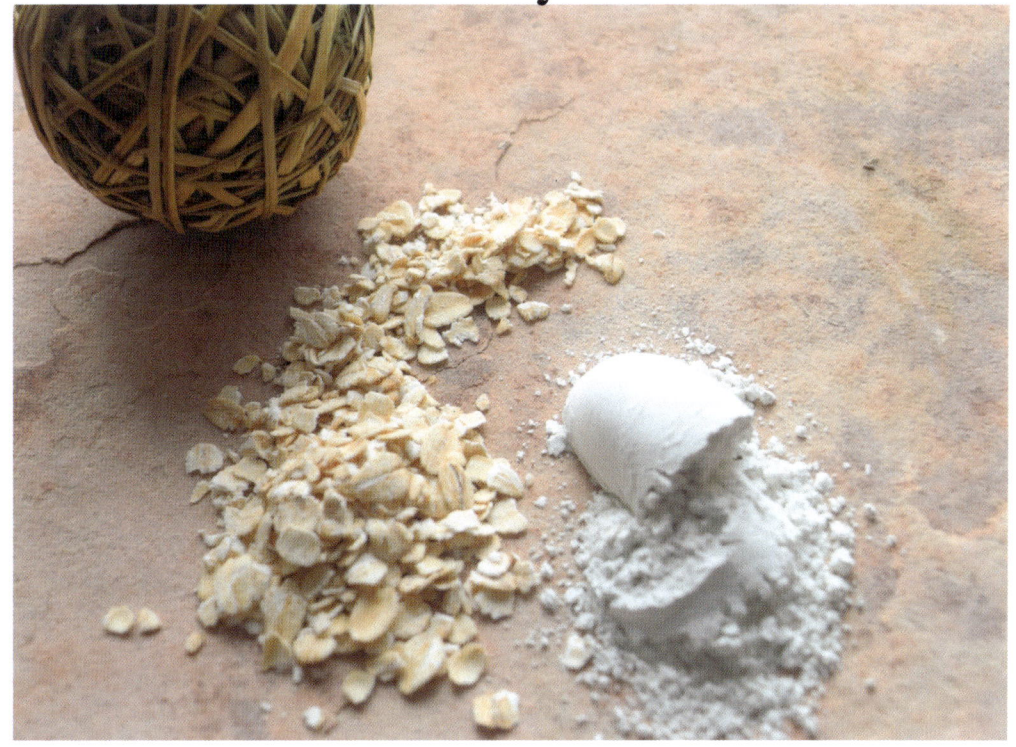

Ingredients:

2 1/2 cups oatmeal (not quick oats)
1/2 cup Bentonite clay
2 tablespoons lemon peel powder
10 drops vitamin E oil
4 drops of lavender essential oil
4 drops of orange essential oil
glass mason jar to store your scrub in

Directions: In a clean coffee grinder or food processor, grind the oats and the lemon peel powder separately until very finely ground. In a bowl mix the ground oatmeal, ground lemon peel powder and Bentonite clay then add the oils and mix well until all is combined. Store in a jar with a lid. This can be stored for up to 6 months.

How to use: In a small bowl add 2-3 tablespoons of water to 2 tablespoons of the scrub mix to form a loose paste and scrub your face gently then rinse.

Benefits: When oatmeal is hydrated it naturally moisturizes and creates a protective barrier on the skin. It also acts as a natural pore cleanser, and is soothing to sensitive skin. Bentonite clay absorbs oils and toxins from the skin's surface. Lemon peel has been known to add a healthy glow and improve skin clarity. It is also believed to be a beneficial part of an acne-prone skin care routine. Vitamin E oil has healing properties. It's an anti-oxidant that helps to deter the effects of free radicals on your skin.

Lavender Body Polish

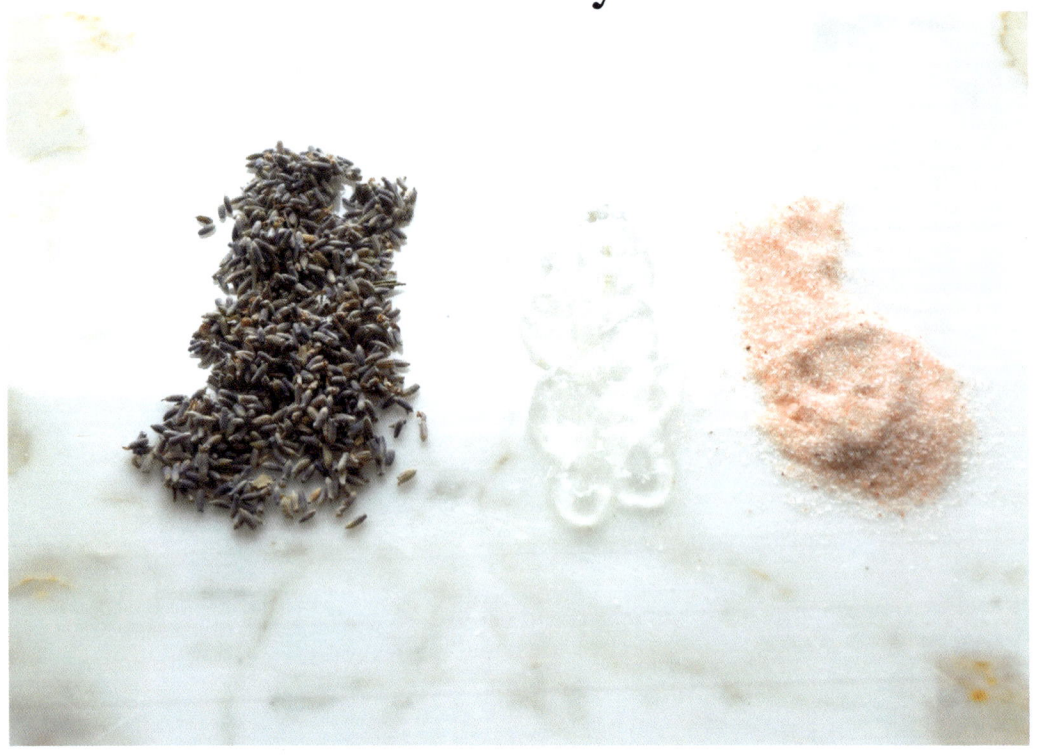

Ingredients:

3 ounces olive oil
1 ounce aloe vera gel
1/2 cup sea salt
1 tablespoon lavender buds ground in a blender or coffee grinder
10 drops of lavender essential oil

Directions:

In a small bowl mix the olive oil, aloe vera gel, and lavender essential oil together. Next add the sea salt and lavender buds powder. Stir the mixture well, making sure to break apart any clumps of salt. After the mixture is thoroughly combined it can be stored in an airtight jar and saved for 7 days.

To use: Take a small amount into the shower and polish your body then rise off. Be careful in the shower the floor may be slippery from the olive oil.

Benefits:

Olive oil's antioxidant properties protect skin cells against environmental damage and inflammation. Aloe vera contains antioxidants, enzymes, vitamins A and C, and it is highly anti-inflammatory. It can help treat burns, acne and dry skin. Lavender essential oil has wonderful healing properties for the skin; it helps relieve itchy skin and acne.

Foot scrub

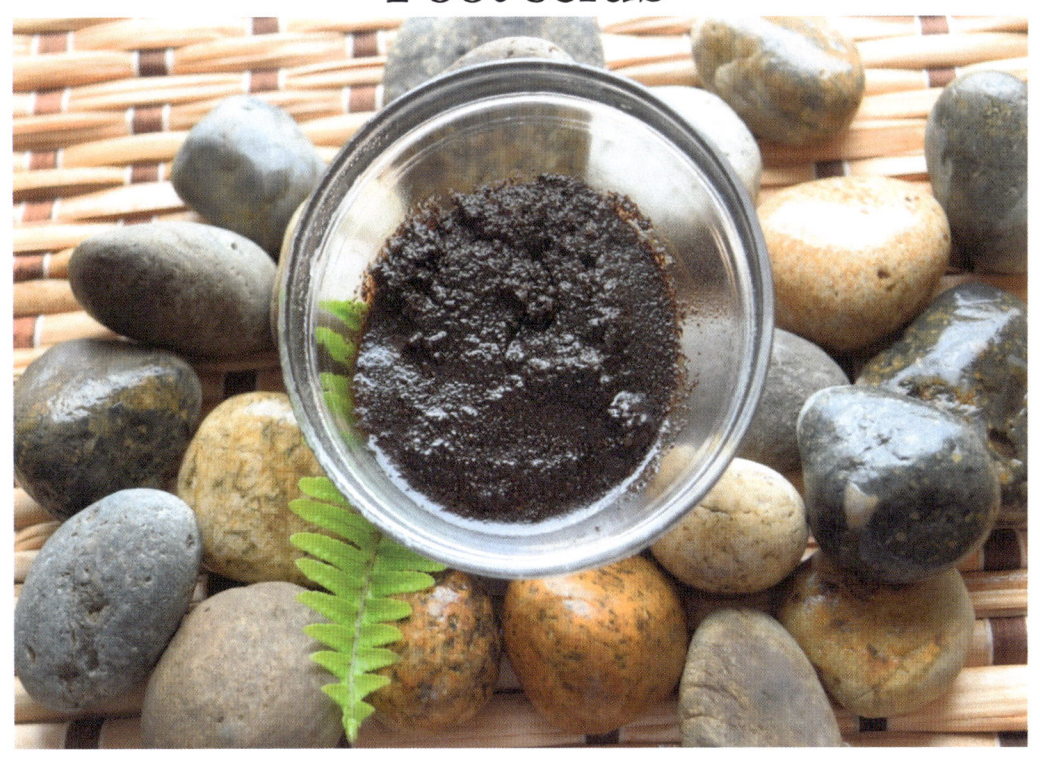

Ingredients:

2 tablespoons sweet almond or apricot kernel oil or olive oil
1 1/2 tablespoons granulated sugar
1 tablespoon ground coffee beans
6 drops sweet orange essential oil
6 drops eucalyptus essential oil

Directions:

Combine all ingredients in a small bowl and mix well.

How to use:

Scoop out a bit of the mixture at a time and scrub feet, working in a circular motion and concentrating on the soles and heels. Rinse with warm water and wipe dry.

Benefits:

Olive oil's antioxidant properties protect skin cells against environmental damage and inflammation. The oil will soften the skin. Coffee is a wonderful gentle exfoliant. Coffee grounds work to gently remove dead skin cells, which helps to rejuvenate and boost circulation. The orange and eucalyptus essential oils have natural antibacterial properties.

Coffee Body Scrub

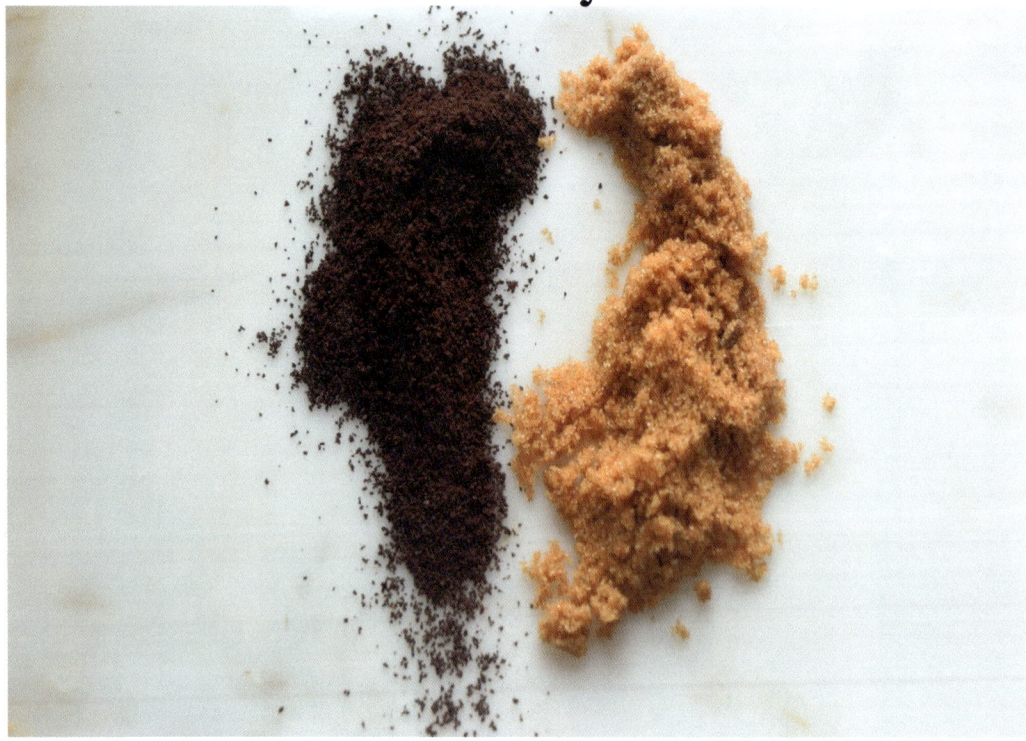

Ingredients:

1/2 cup fresh ground coffee (choose fine grounds, as the coarse kind can be too harsh for sensitive or delicate skin.)
1/2 cup brown sugar
1/2 cup melted coconut oil
1 teaspoon vanilla extract

Directions:

Mix together the fresh ground coffee and brown sugar. Add the coconut oil into the coffee mixture and 1 tsp. vanilla extract. Mix until well until combined.

To use:

Gently rub the mixture over your body in the shower avoid areas around the eyes. Rinse thoroughly. (Be careful if using the scrub in the shower, the oil can make the floor a bit slippery.)

Benefits:

Coffee is a wonderful gentle exfoliant. Applying coffee directly to your skin may help decrease the appearance of sun spots, redness, and fine lines. The sand-like texture of coffee grounds makes a great exfoliant in homemade scrubs. The grounds work to gently remove dead skin cells, which helps to rejuvenate and boost circulation. Coconut oil may be linked to some potential benefits for skin, including reducing inflammation, keeping skin moisturized and helping heal wounds. The medium-chain fatty acids found in coconut oil also possess antimicrobial properties that can help treat acne and protect the skin from harmful bacteria. The brown sugar is a natural gentle exfoliant.

Summer Body Scrub

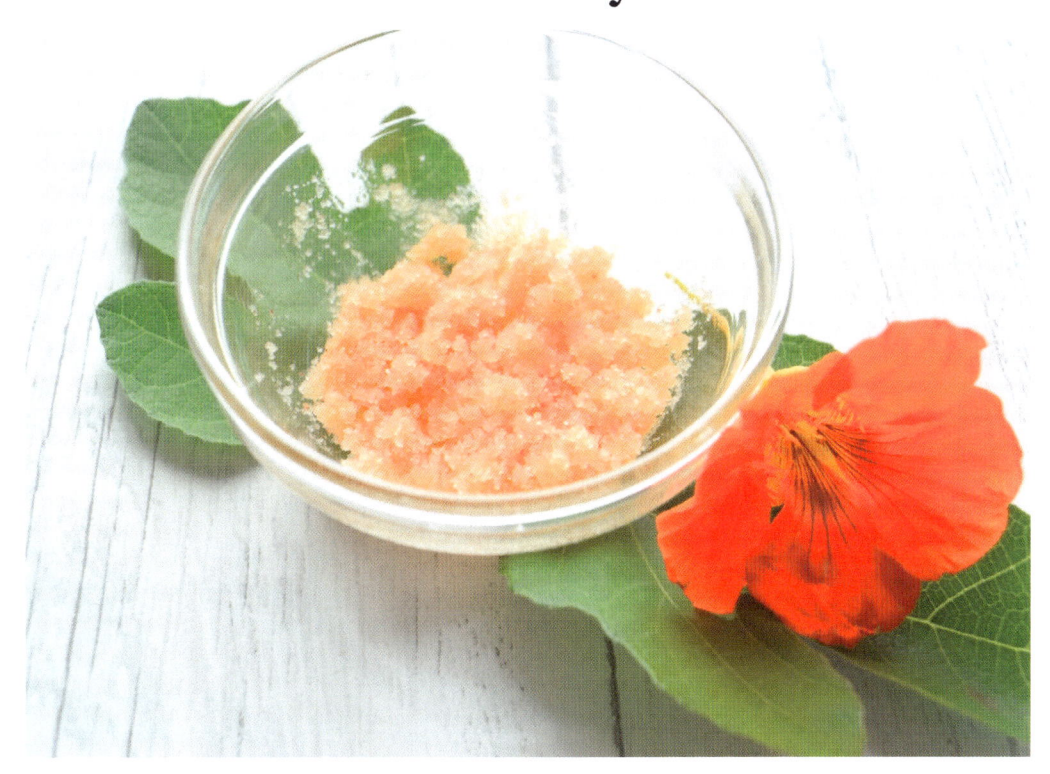

Ingredients:

1/2 cup fine grain natural salt or sugar
1-2 ounces olive oil
10 drops of either lavender, grapefruit, orange, or geranium essential oil

Directions:

Mix salt/sugar with olive oil in a bowl then add the essential oil. This should be used within a day or two. Store in an airtight container.

To use:

Take a small amount into your hand and polish your body while you are in the shower, then rise off. Be careful your shower may become slippery because of the olive oil.

Benefits:

This super quick scrub works really well to soften your skin and exfoliate leaving your skin nice and smooth. The salt and sugar are natural gentle exfoliants that will not cause skin irritation. Olive oil's antioxidant properties protect skin cells against environmental damage and inflammation. Lavender essential oil has wonderful healing properties for the skin; it helps relieve itchy skin and acne. Grapefruit essential oil is a natural anti-inflammatory. The essential oil of grapefruit is said to be an anti-depressant because it has a cheering and refreshing fragrance. Grapefruit essential oil has natural antibacterial and astringent properties. It may help with acne and oily skin.

Lip Scrub

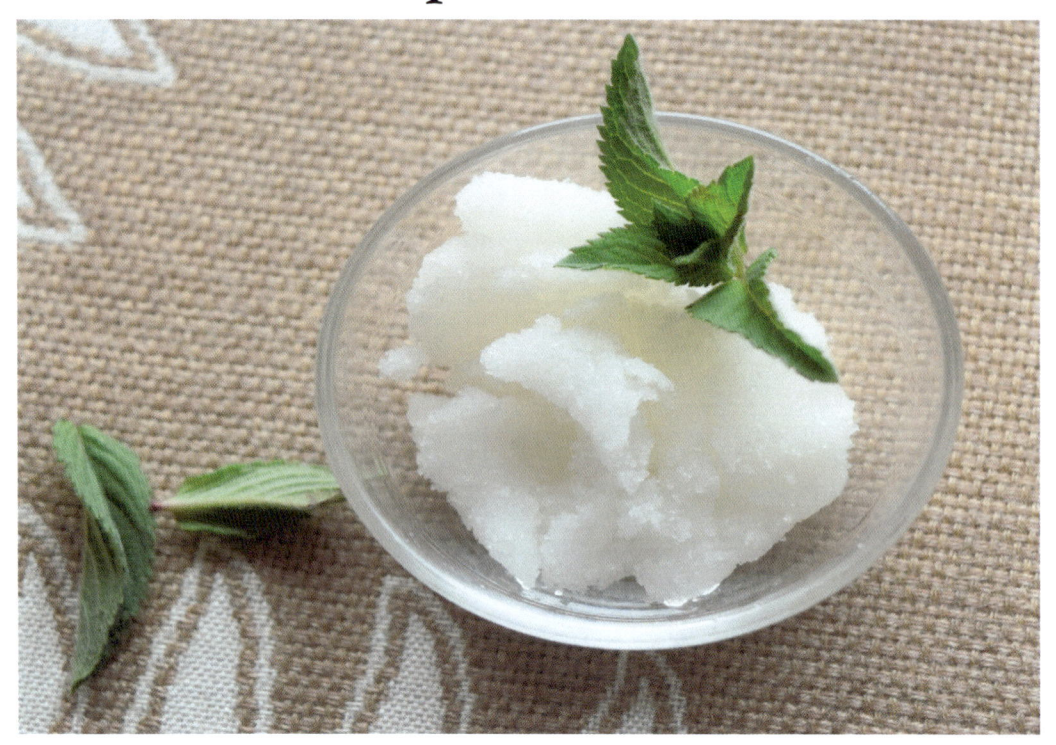

Ingredients:

2 drops of peppermint oil the edible type (you can get it at your local grocery store in the bakery aisle)
1 tablespoon of sugar
1 tablespoon of coconut oil

Directions:

Place sugar and coconut oil in a bowl and add the peppermint oil and mix well. You can keep this in the refrigerator for 1 week.

To use:

Scoop out a small amount with your finger, and then gently rub the mixture over your lips. Then rise off.

Benefits:

The sugar gently removes dry skin from your lips and the coconut oil will soften them. Coconut oil may be linked to some potential benefits for skin, including reducing inflammation, keeping skin moisturized and helping heal wounds. The medium-chain fatty acids found in coconut oil also possess antimicrobial properties.

Honey and Olive Oil Hair Conditioner

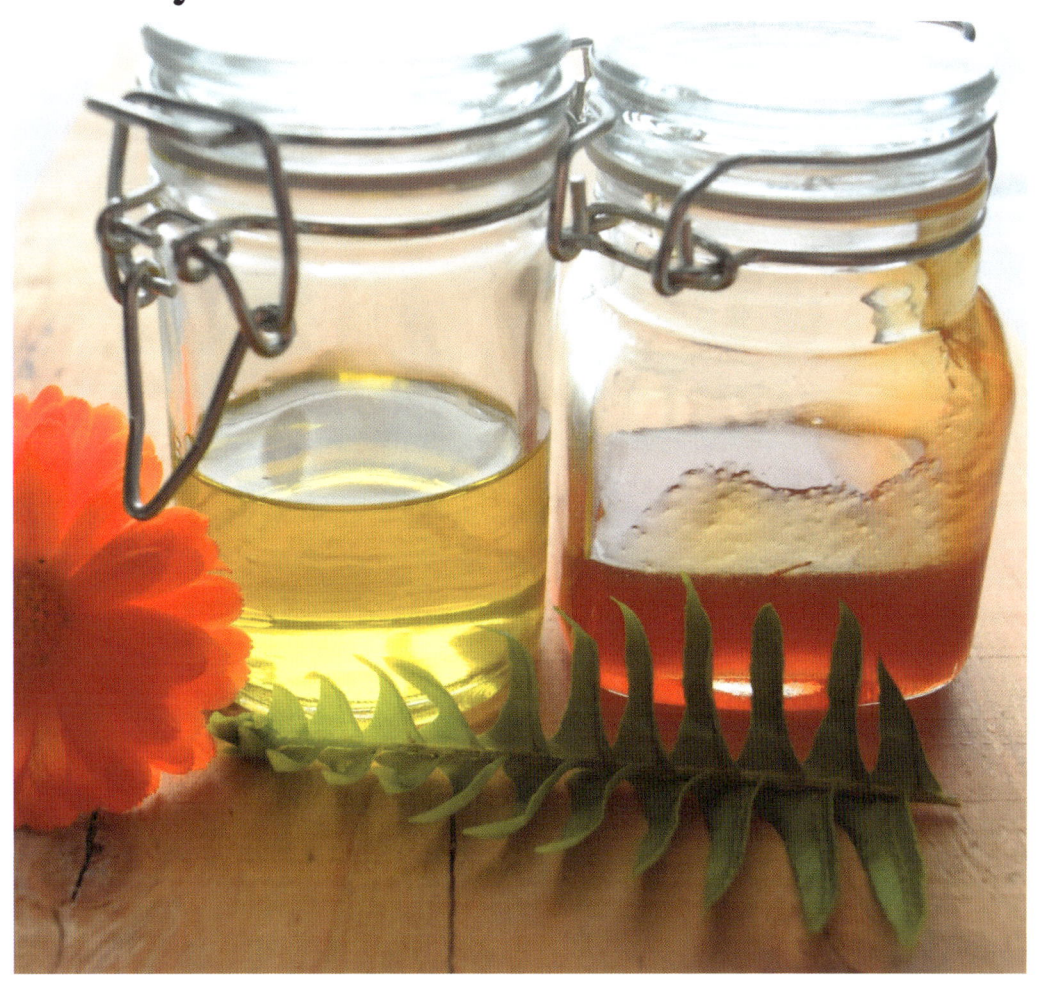

Ingredients:

2 tablespoons of honey
4 tablespoons of olive oil
shower cap

Directions: In a bowl combine the honey and olive oil until you get a smooth mixture.

How to use:

Divide your hair into four sections and start applying the mixture to it with a clean paint brush or your hands. Once your hair is fully covered put the shower cap on and leave on for 30 minutes. Then wash your hair. You can use this once or twice a month.

Benefits:

Olive oil's antioxidant properties protect skin cells against environmental damage and inflammation. Olive oil will soften your hair and nourish it. Honey has antibacterial and antiseptic properties, so it gets rid of dirt and bacteria. It's full of antioxidants and boosts collagen production. It's extremely moisturizing and hydrates even the driest of skin. Honey is naturally soothing and has healing properties. It also works as a clarifying agent.

Shea Butter & Coconut Oil Hair Conditioner

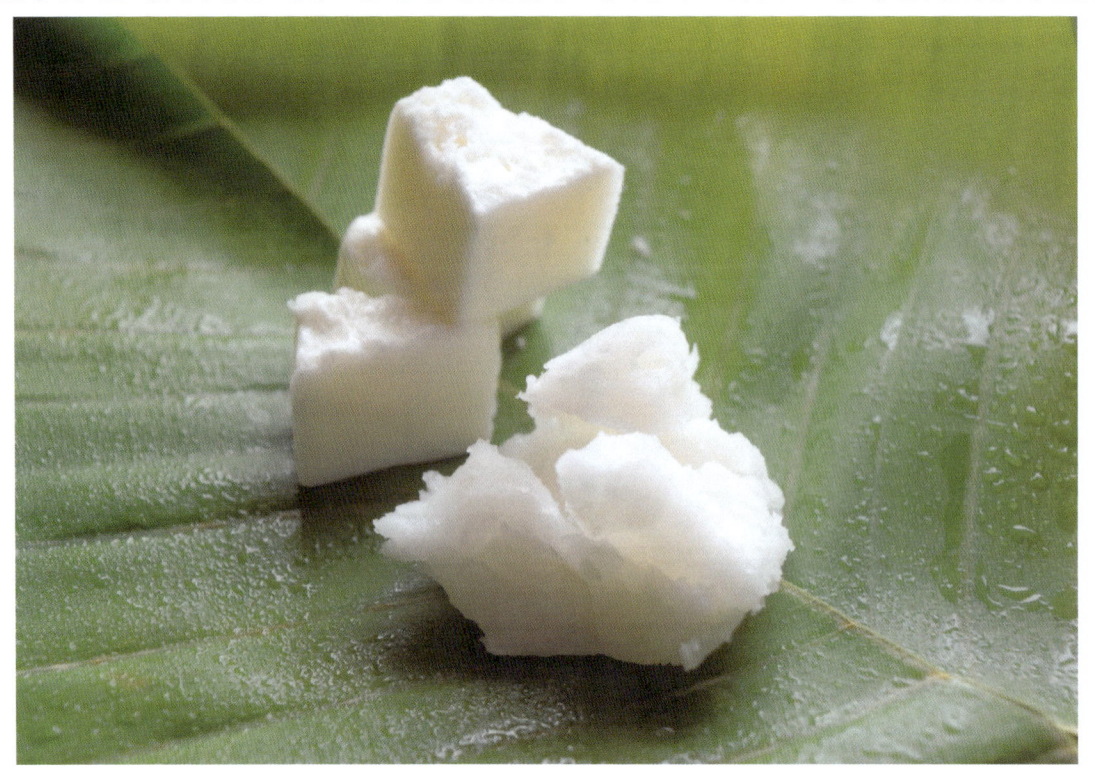

Ingredients:

1 tablespoon shea butter
2 tablespoons coconut oil
1 teaspoon argan oil
2-3 drops of an essential oil of your choice (optional)

Directions:

Put the shea butter and coconut oil in a small glass container and melt slowly in the microwave, do 20 seconds at a time until melted. Then add the argan oil and essential oil. Mix well.

How to use:

Put a small amount into your hands and apply to your hair until all of your hair is covered. Leave on for 30 minutes then wash your hair as usual. You can use this 2-3 times a month.

Benefits:

Shea butter is an abundant source of fatty acids and oils. It is rich in vitamin C and has antioxidant and anti-inflammatory. Shea butter is widely used as a conditioner, especially for curly hair. Coconut oil may be linked to some potential benefits for skin and hair keeping hair moisturized and soft. The medium-chain fatty acids found in coconut oil also possess antimicrobial properties. Coconut oil is an amazing moisturizer.

Toothpaste #1

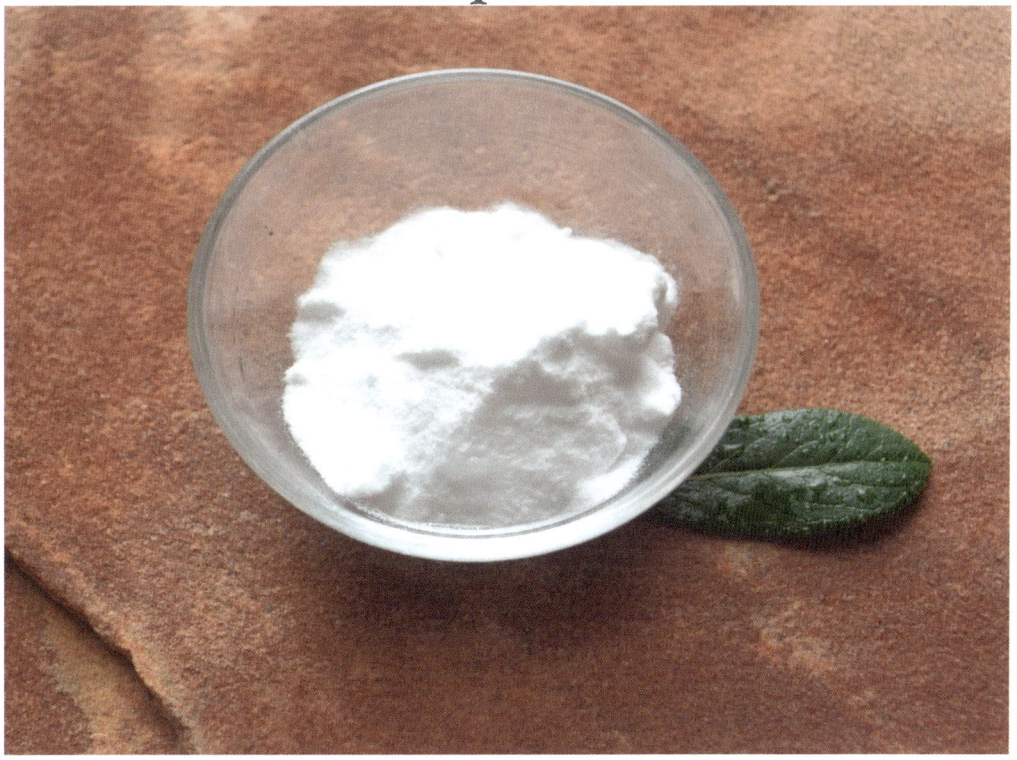

Toothpaste with baking soda and water

1 teaspoon baking soda
add a few drops of water

Toothpaste with baking soda, salt and water

1 tablespoon baking soda
1 tablespoon of natural salt
add three drops of peppermint essential oil
add a few drops of water

Toothpaste with baking soda and coconut oil

2 tablespoon baking soda
2 tablespoon of coconut oil
3 drops of peppermint essential oil

Directions: Mix all the ingredients well to get a smooth texture.

How to use: Dip your toothbrush in the mixture and brush your teeth.

Benefits:

There are other benefits of brushing your teeth with baking soda apart from just a brighter smile. By attacking the plaque formation it prevents dental decay, cavity formation and gum diseases to a very large extent. It also fights bad breath by balancing the acidic levels of residual food.

Toothpaste #2

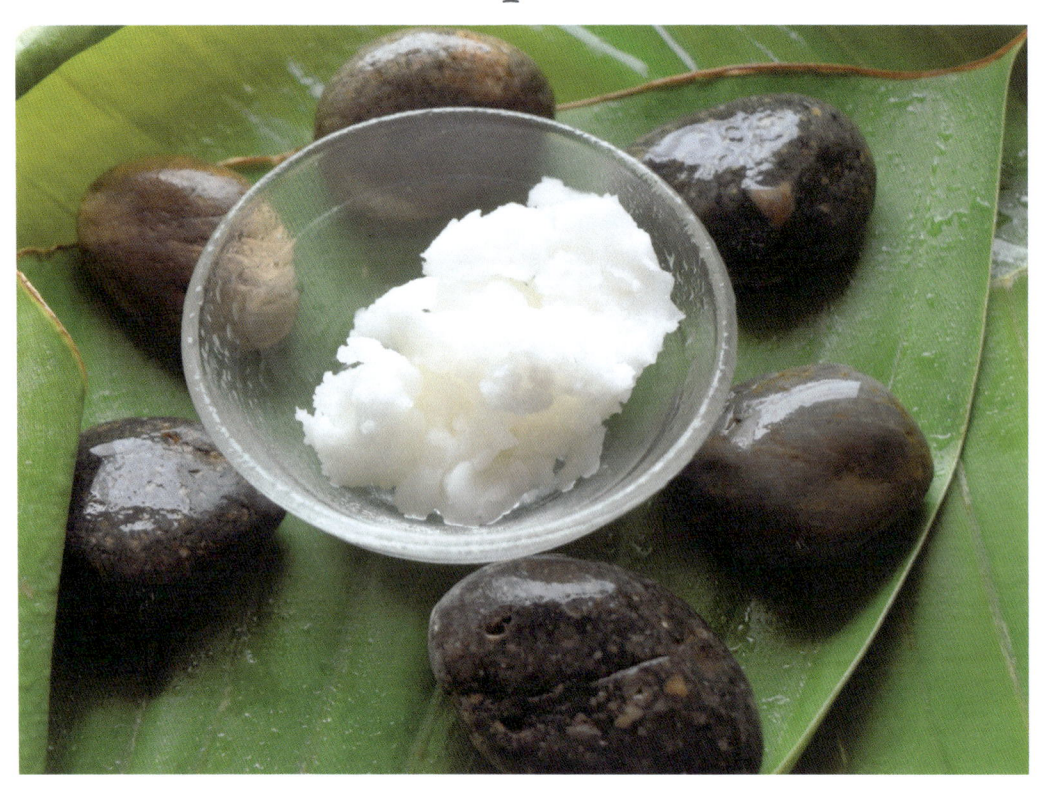

Ingredients:

1/2 cup coconut oil
2-3 tablespoons of baking soda
1 small packet stevia powder
10 drops peppermint oil (you can find peppermint oil in the bakery aisle at your grocery store)

Directions:

Slightly soften the coconut oil in the microwave for 20 seconds in a small glass container. Mix in other ingredients and stir well. Let cool completely. Store in an airtight container.

To use:

Add a small amount to toothbrush then brush your teeth.

Benefits:

There are other benefits of brushing your teeth with baking soda apart from just a brighter smile. By attacking the plaque formation it prevents dental decay, cavity formation and gum diseases to a very large extent. It also fights bad breath by balancing the acidic levels of residual food. The coconut acts as a carrier for the baking soda and the peppermint gives it a refreshing flavor.

Dry Shampoo #1

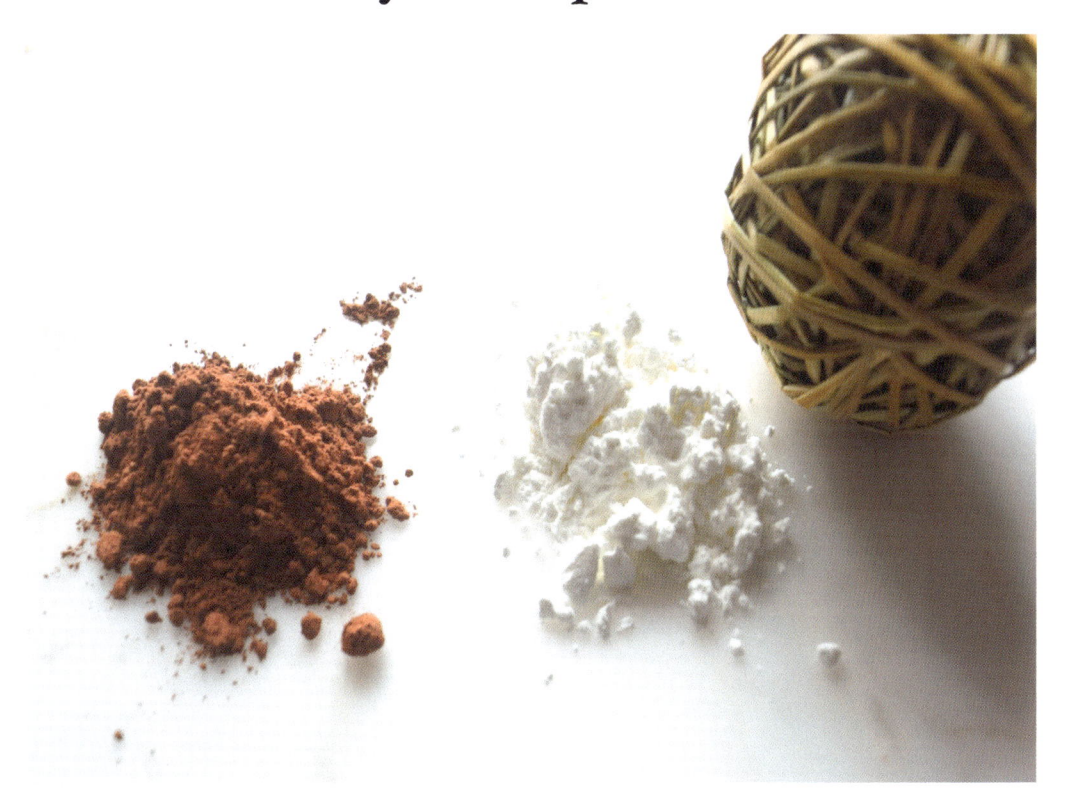

Ingredients:

1/4 cup arrowroot powder
(for dark hair use 2 tablespoons of arrowroot and 1 tablespoon of cocoa powder)
5 drops of an essential oil that you like

Directions:

Place the arrowroot, or arrowroot and cocoa powder, into a small jar. Add the essential oil and mix to combine.

How to use:

Apply with a make-up brush to the roots or oily parts of your hair. Then brush out your hair.

Benefits:

The arrowroot will draw out the oils in your hair. If you have dark hair the cocoa powder will make the mixture dark and not show up in your hair if there is any left behind after you brush out your hair. The arrowroot can make hair softer, smoother, and less oily since it absorbs excess oil it may add some body too.

Dry Shampoo #2

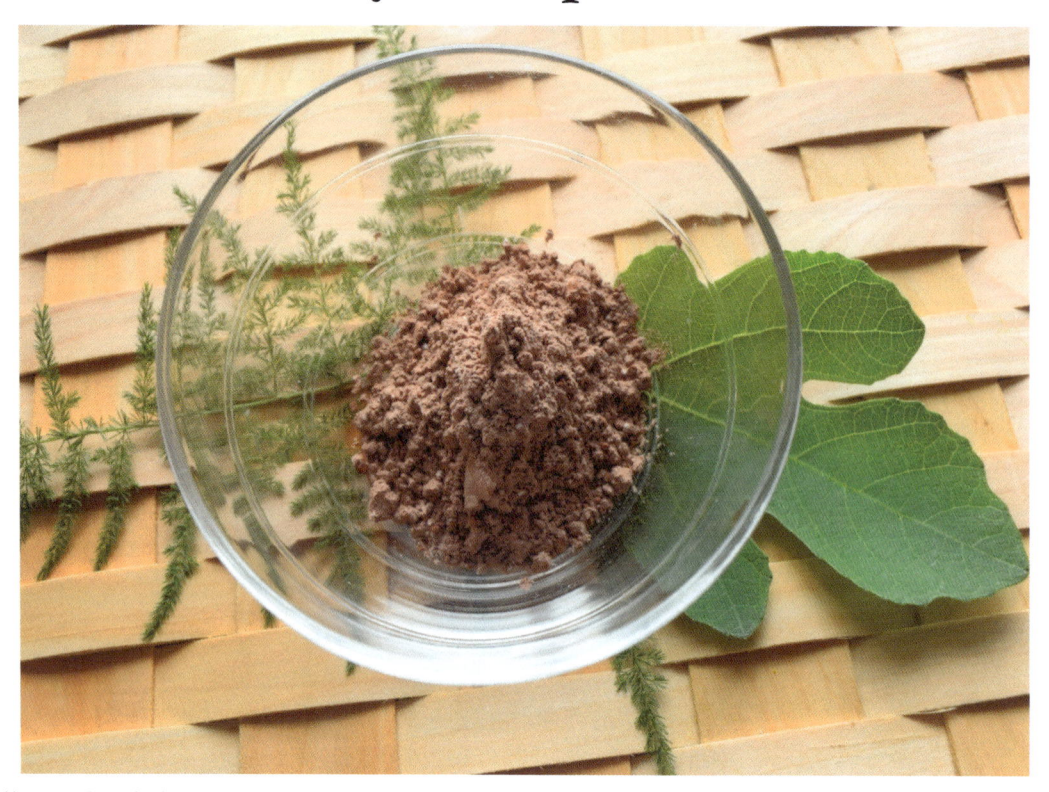

Ingredients for light hair:

1/4 cup corn starch
1 tablespoon baking soda
5 drops of your favorite essential oil

Directions: Combine the corn starch and baking soda and essential oil together in a small bowl. Mix well and transfer to a small container with a lid. Use a makeup brush to apply to your roots then brush out.

Ingredients for dark hair:

1/4 cup corn starch
1 tablespoon baking soda
1 tablespoon cocoa powder
5 drops of your favorite essential oil.

Directions: Combine the corn starch, cocoa powder, baking soda and essential oil together in a small bowl. Mix well and transfer to a small container with a lid. Use a makeup brush to apply to your roots then brush out.

Benefits:

The corn starch will draw out the oils in your hair. If you have dark hair the cocoa powder will make the mixture dark and not show up in your hair if there is any left behind after you brush out your hair. The corn starch can make hair softer, smoother, and less oily since it absorbs excess oil.

Shampoo Bar

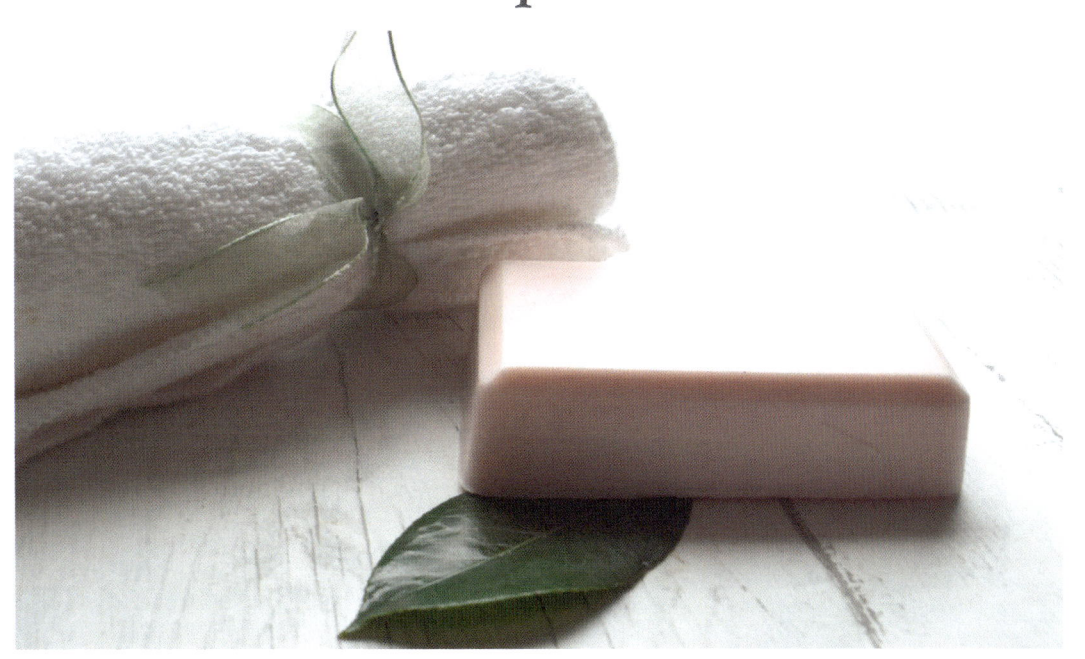

Ingredients:

1 lb of Melt and Pour Shaving Soap Base (from Bulk Apothecary)
1 teaspoon almond oil
2 tablespoons of shea butter
1 teaspoon of French pink clay
2-3 drops rosemary essential oil
2-3 drops lemon essential oil
2-3 drops grapefruit essential oil
silicon mold such as for cupcakes or ice cubes

Directions:

Combine the oils and shea butter and melt them in a glass bowl and melt slowly on low in the microwave. Keep them warm while you melt the soap base in a double boiler. Melt the soap base on medium, do not let it boil. When the soap has melted add the butters, oils, clay, and then add the essential oils Gently mix until all is combined. Pour into silicon molds that is on a cookie sheet (it is easier to move the mold) and let harden and completely cool about 4 hours.

To use:

Get the soap and your hair wet you can rub the bar directly onto your hair or lather it up in your hands then add to your hair. Rinse and repeat if necessary. Makes 4, 4 oz. bars.

Benefits:

Rosemary stimulates circulation which can be good for hair growth. Shea butter provides moisture to dry or damaged hair from the roots to the very tips, repairing and protecting against weather damage, dryness and brittleness. It also absorbs quickly and completely into the scalp to rehydrate without clogging pores. It is particularly beneficial for processed and heat-treated hair.

Coconut Oil Lotion Bars

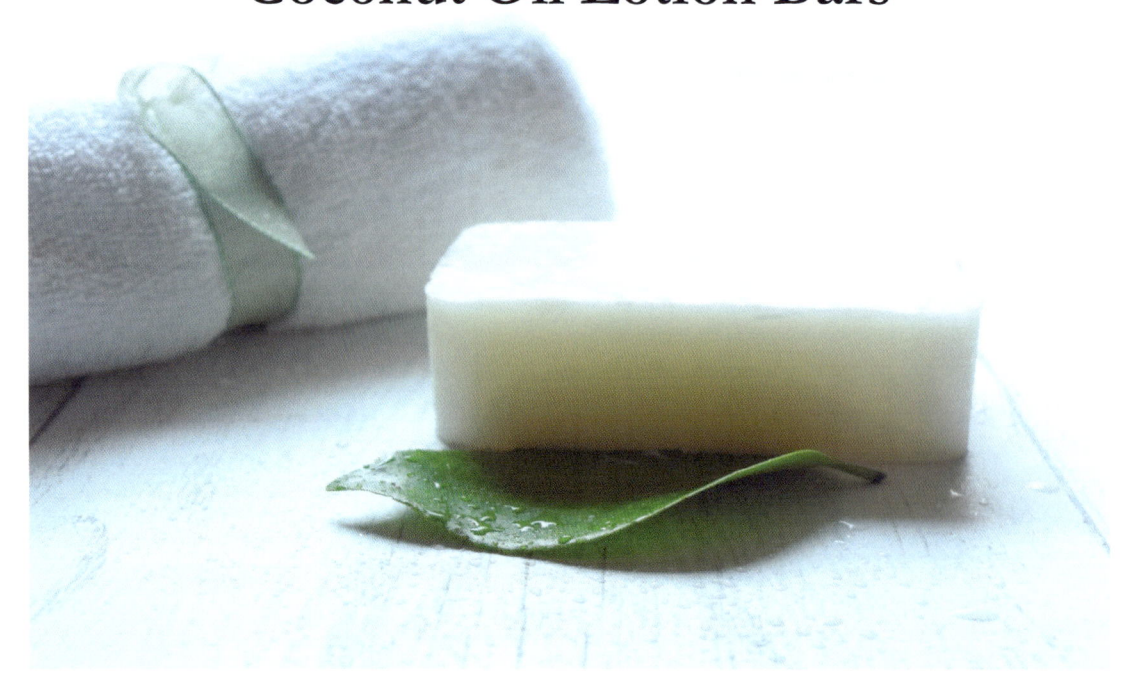

Ingredients:

1 cup coconut oil
1 cup beeswax pellets
1/2 cup shea butter
1/2 cup almond oil
10 drops of essential oil of your choice
silicon mold such as for cupcakes or ice cubes

Directions:

Place all ingredients except essential oils in a double boiler combine the coconut oil and beeswax, shea butter, melt on low heat stir regularly until all ingredients melt completely. Let cool slightly. Add essential oils and almond oil. Stir to combine all of the ingredients. Pour the mix into silicone molds that is on a cookie sheet (it makes it easier to move the mold) Let set completely 4-6 hours. Pop out of the molds and store in an air tight container.

To use:

Rub onto your skin and rub it in, that's it!

Benefits:

High concentrations of fatty acids and vitamins make shea butter an ideal cosmetic ingredient for softening skin. Shea butter also has anti-inflammatory and healing properties. Using shea butter on your body can condition, tone, and soothe your skin. Coconut oil may be linked to some potential benefits for skin, including reducing inflammation, keeping skin moisturized and helping heal wounds. The medium-chain fatty acids found in coconut oil also possess antimicrobial properties that can help treat acne and protect the skin from harmful bacteria. Almond oil treats dry skin. It improves acne and it helps reverse sun damage.

Bath Tub Tea

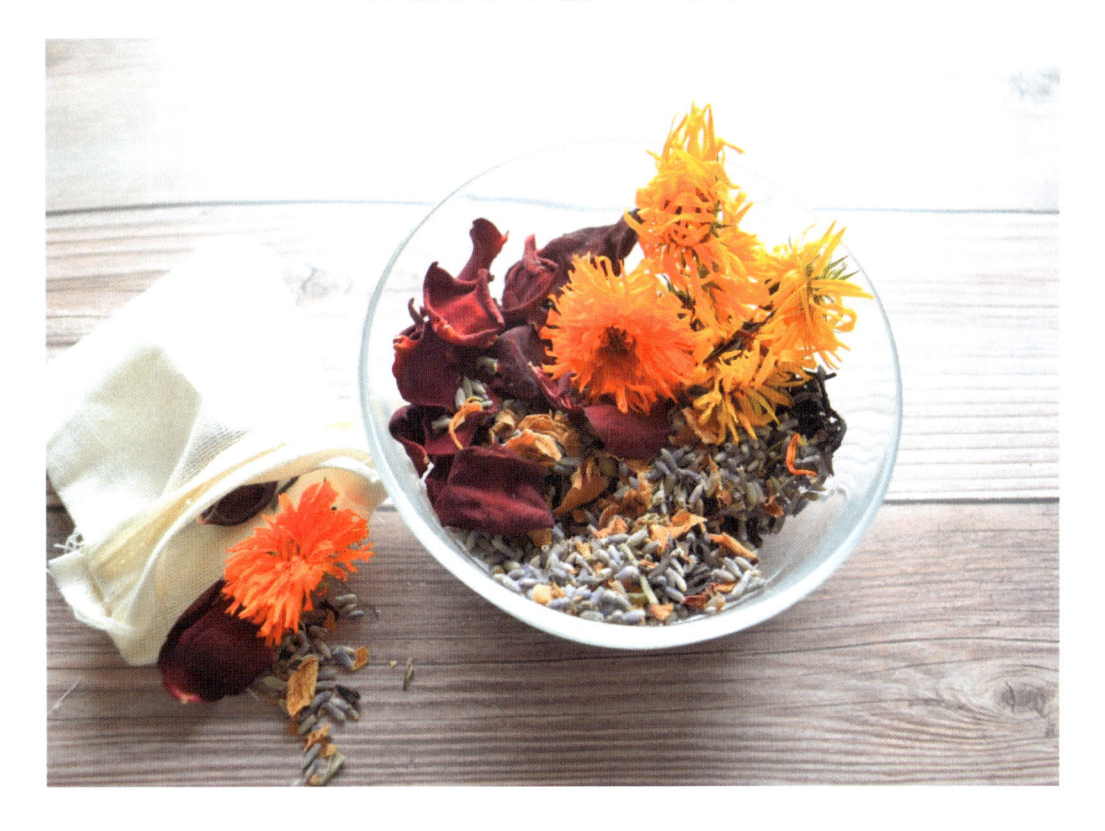

Ingredients:

1/4 cup dried lavender buds
1/4 cup dried chamomile buds
1/4 cup dried rose petals
1/4 cup dried hibiscus petals
1/4 cup dried Calendula flowers
muslin bag
A mason jar with a lid to store your tub tea in.

Directions: Mix all together in a large bowl. Store in an airtight container.

To use: Put a scoop of tea in a muslin bag and run under warm bath water and enjoy.

Benefits:

There is something wonderful about soaking in a warm tub with botanicals. It revives your spirits. Lavender is very aromatic and herbaceous, slightly sweet. Lavender has wonderful healing properties for the skin; it helps relieve itchy skin and acne. Lavender has natural antibacterial and antidepressant properties. Chamomile has wonderful skin healing properties, which include helping to tone skin, it is good for rashes, and it softens the skin and acts as an anti-inflammatory. Chamomile is also good for sensitive skin. It is calming and soothing. Rose also has anti-inflammatory properties, which means it can be put on the skin to soothe irritation. Rose has antiseptic and antibacterial properties; it can help wounds heal faster by keeping them clean and fighting infections. Hibiscus can encourage an all round fresher, younger, smoother looking skin. The natural acids present in hibiscus help to purify your skin by breaking down dead skin and increasing cell turnover, it can even help to control acne breakouts.

Milk Bath

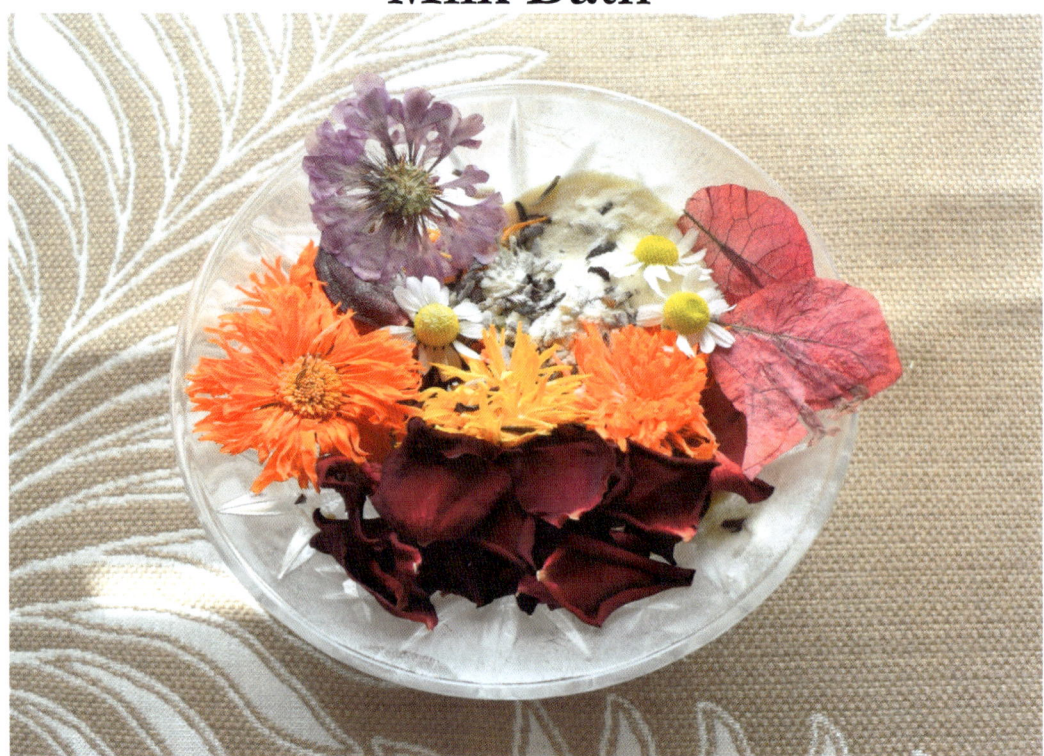

Ingredients:

2 cups milk powder (non-fat dry milk works)
1 cup oat flour or rice flour finely ground (you can grind your own)
1/2 cup of herbs such as lavender, chamomile or rose petals
1/4 cup of baking soda
2–4 teaspoons of essential oil of your choice chamomile and lavender work well.

Directions: Mix all ingredients in a large bowl. Store in an air tight container.

To Use: Put a scoop of milk bath in a muslin bag run under warm bath water. Soak until the water cools.

Benefits:

This soothing skin friendly bath soak will relax you and nourish your skin.

Lavender is very aromatic and herbaceous, slightly sweet. Lavender essential oil has wonderful healing properties for the skin; it helps relieve itchy skin and acne. Lavender has natural antibacterial and antidepressant properties. The fragrance revives your spirits. Chamomile has wonderful skin healing properties, which include helping to tone skin, it is good for rashes, and it softens the skin and acts as an anti-inflammatory. Chamomile is also good for sensitive skin. It is calming and soothing. Rose also has anti-inflammatory properties, which means it can be put on the skin to soothe irritation. Rose has antiseptic and antibacterial properties; it can help wounds heal faster, by keeping them clean and fighting infections. A milk bath leaves your skin feeling soft and supple. The acid in the milk also helps exfoliate the skin for additional softness. The lactic acid in milk helps clean and soften the skin.

After Shave

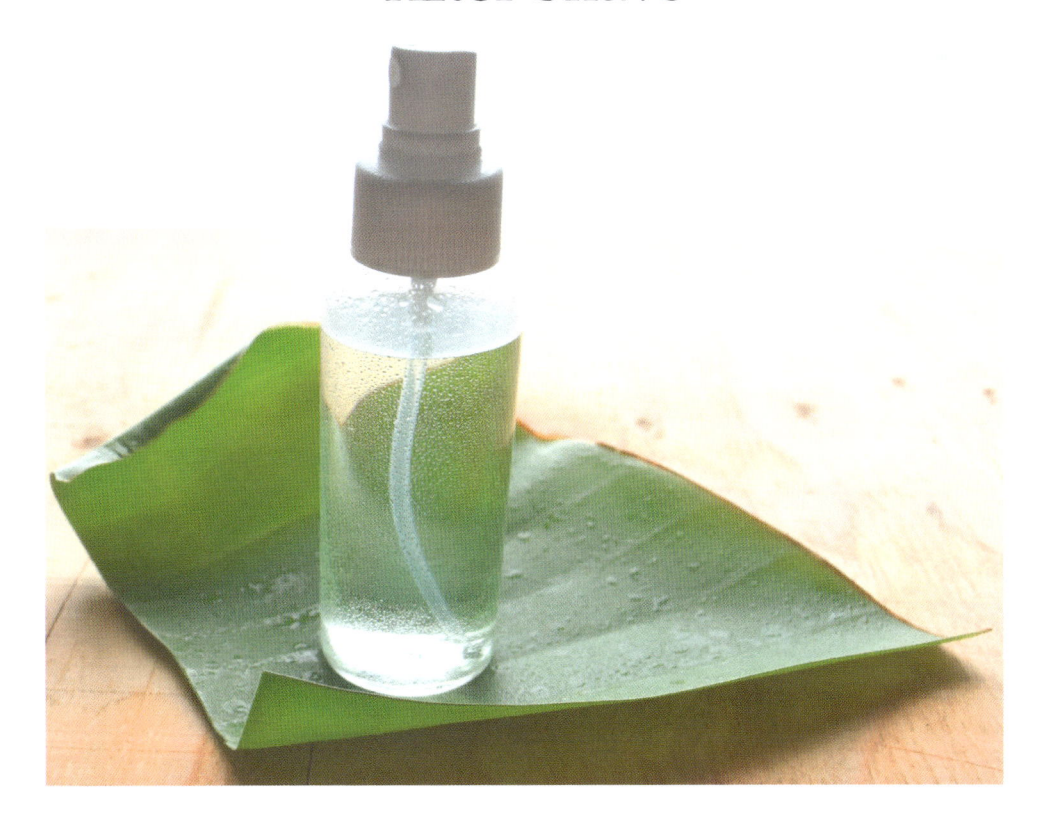

Ingredients:

1 oz of distilled water
1 oz witch hazel
1/4 teaspoon of vegetable glycerin
1/4 teaspoon jojoba oil

13 drops of cedar wood essential oil
10 drops of lime essential oil
2 drops of vitamin E oil
Small bottle to store your after shave in.

Directions: Add glycerin, jojoba oil, essential oils and vitamin E to the spray bottle. Add the water and then fill rest of the way with witch hazel. Shake until well combined.

To use: Shake well and spray on hands then apply to face or spray your face directly avoid your eyes and mouth.

Benefits: This great smelling aftershave is wonderful for your skin with the nourishing jojoba oil and glycerin. Witch hazel is a plant that is native to North America, the bark and leaves are used to make a skin healing astringent. Glycerin acts like a sponge and draws moisture from the air to your skin. It also helps slow down the evaporation of water from the skin, which can help keep skin moist and hydrated. Cedar wood essential oil may help with oily skin and acne as well as eczema. Cedar essential oil also has antiseptic properties. Lime essential oil has natural anti-microbial, antiseptic and astringent actions. It is a natural antioxidant. It is detoxifying, and may help with oily skin, or acne.

Peppermint Foot Balm

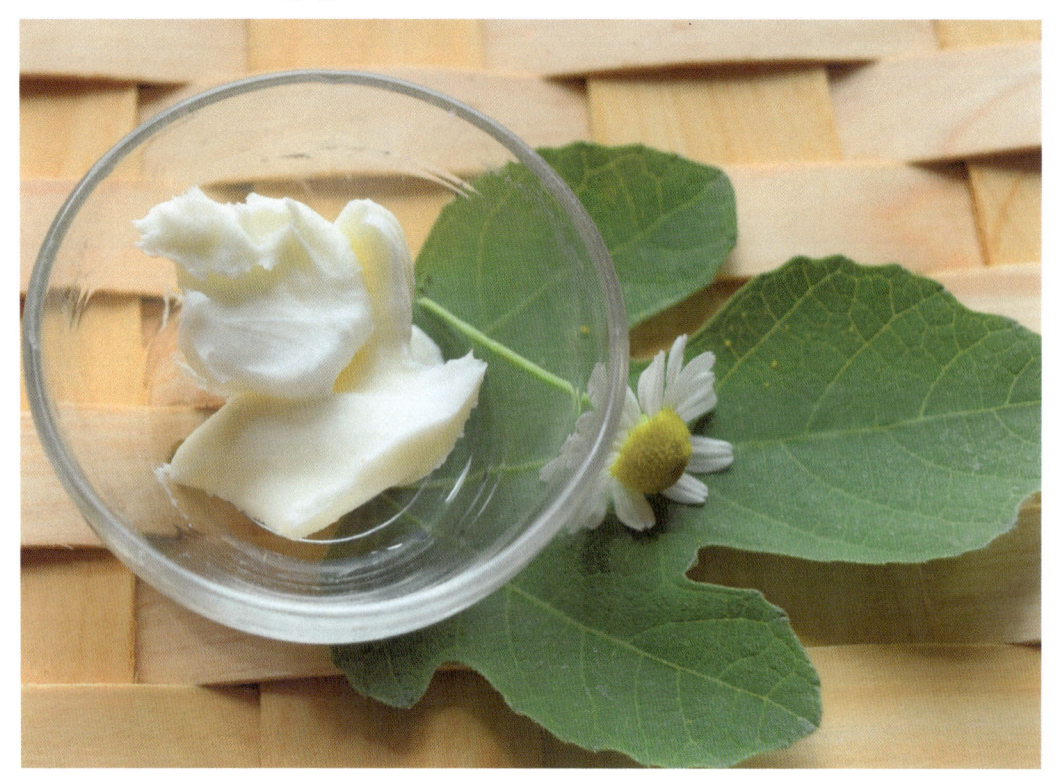

Ingredients:

1/4 cup olive oil
1/4 cup coconut oil
1/4 cup cocoa butter
1 tablespoon of grated beeswax or bees wax pellets
25 drops peppermint essential oil
5 drops tea tree essential oil
small jar with a lid

Directions:

Melt the oils, wax and cocoa butter together over medium-low heat in a double boiler. Add essential oils when the oils and wax are melted. Pour into a small glass jar with a lid and leave undisturbed for 6-8 hours to cool.

To use: Rub into your feet and put some socks on so you don't slip on the floor!

Benefits:

Olive oil's antioxidant properties protect skin cells against environmental damage and inflammation. Coconut oil may be linked to some potential benefits for skin, including reducing inflammation, keeping skin moisturized and helping heal wounds. The medium-chain fatty acids found in coconut oil also possess antimicrobial properties that can help treat acne and protect the skin from harmful bacteria. Peppermint essential oil has anti-inflammatory and astringent properties. It's vitalizing and refreshing it energizes the mind and body. Mint also helps clean pores. It has a powerful sweet crisp scent. It relieves muscle and joint pain. It also has cooling, invigorating and antispasmodic properties. Tea Tree essential oil has natural antibacterial properties.

Cuticle Oil

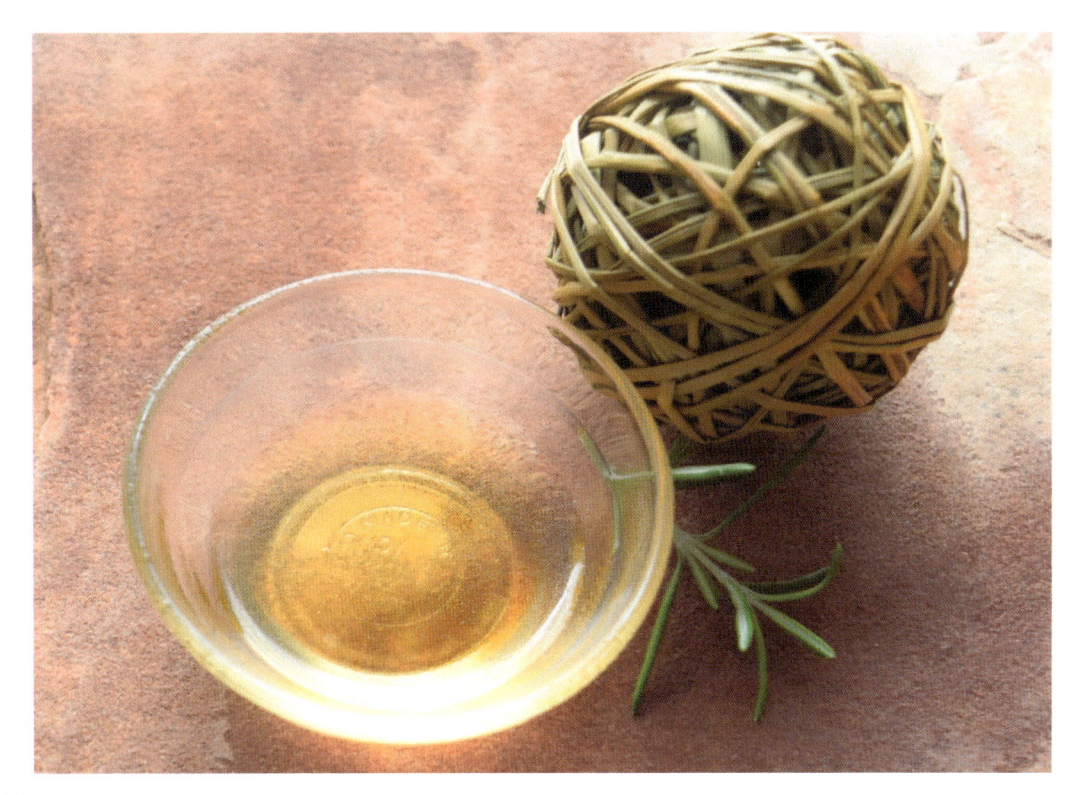

Ingredients:

3 teaspoon olive oil
1/2 teaspoon avocado oil
1 tablespoon jojoba oil
12 drops lavender essential oil
12 drops rosemary essential oil
12 drops lemon essential oil
small glass jar with a lid

Directions: In a small glass bowl combine all the ingredients and mix well. Transfer to a small jar with a lid.

How to use:

Add one drop to each nail and massage in. Keep it on for 15 minutes then wash your hands with soap and water. You can use this once a week.

Benefits:

Olive oil's antioxidant properties protect skin cells against environmental damage and inflammation. Olive oil will also make your skin soft. Avocado oil contains a high percentage of vitamin E, as well as potassium, lecithin, and many other nutrients which can nourish and moisturize your skin. The oleic acid also promotes collagen production, which helps grow new skin. Lavender essential oil has natural antibacterial properties. Rosemary essential oil can help circulation and is a natural antioxidant. It is very invigorating. Lemon essential oil may help to detoxify skin.

Cuticle Softener

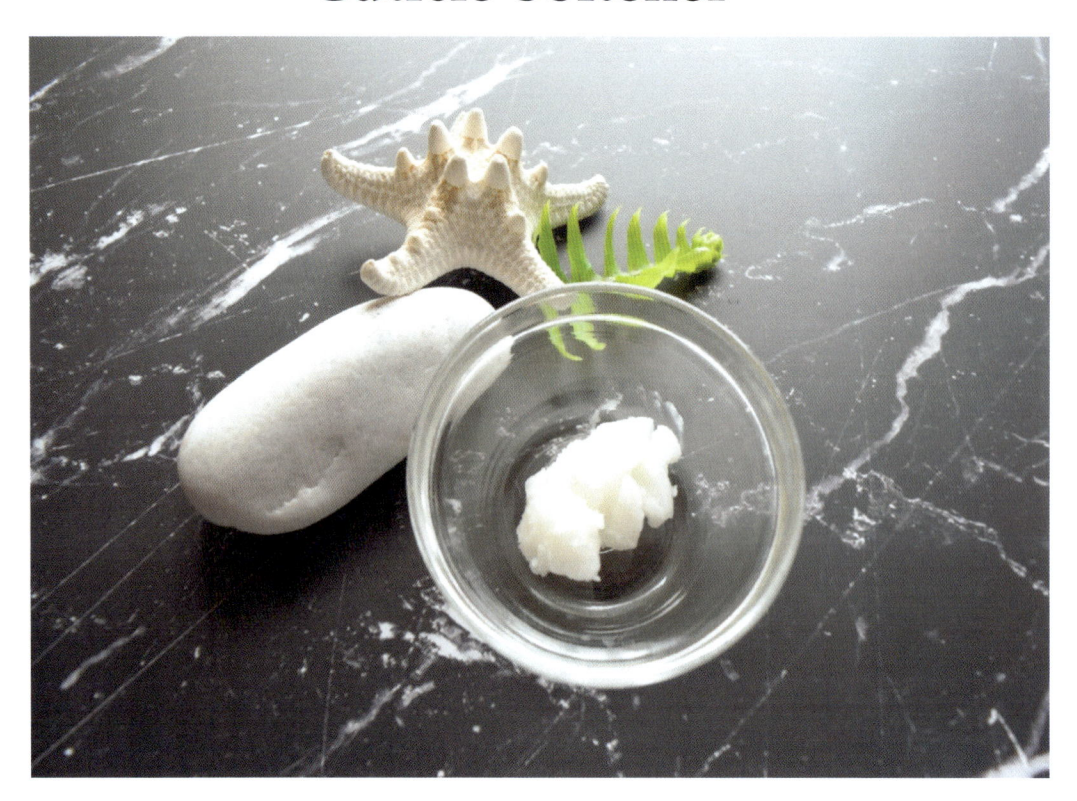

Ingredients:

2 tablespoons of coconut oil
2 drops of geranium essential oil
small jar with a lid

Directions:

Mix the ingredients completely then store in a small jar with a lid.

How to use:

Rub a small amount onto each nail. You can use this once a week.

Benefits:

Coconut oil may be linked to some potential benefits for skin, including reducing inflammation, keeping skin moisturized and helping heal wounds. The medium-chain fatty acids found in coconut oil also possess antimicrobial properties. Geranium is reputed to effectively eliminate dead cells, tighten the skin, promote the regeneration of new skin, and diminish signs of aging.

Finger Nail Soak

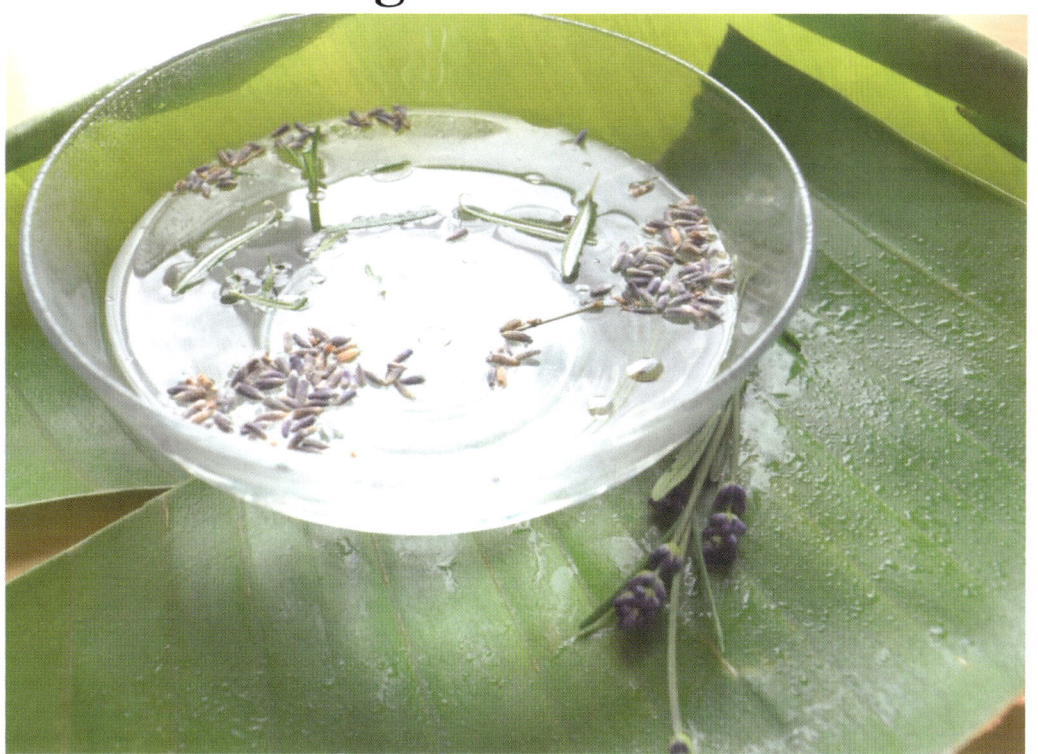

Ingredients:

1 cup of warm water
1 teaspoon of dried ground lavender buds
1/2 teaspoon of dried rosemary
1 teaspoon of lemon juice
1 teaspoon of olive oil

Directions:

Put the water in a small bowl that both your hands will fit into. Add the lavender buds, rosemary, lemon juice and olive oil and stir until blended.

How to use:

Soak your finger nails in the warm solution for 15 minutes.

Benefits:

Olive oil's antioxidant properties protect skin cells against environmental damage and inflammation. Olive oil will also make your skin soft. The lemon essential oil is purifying and the rosemary stimulates circulation. Lavender is a natural antibacterial agent.

Natural Deodorant

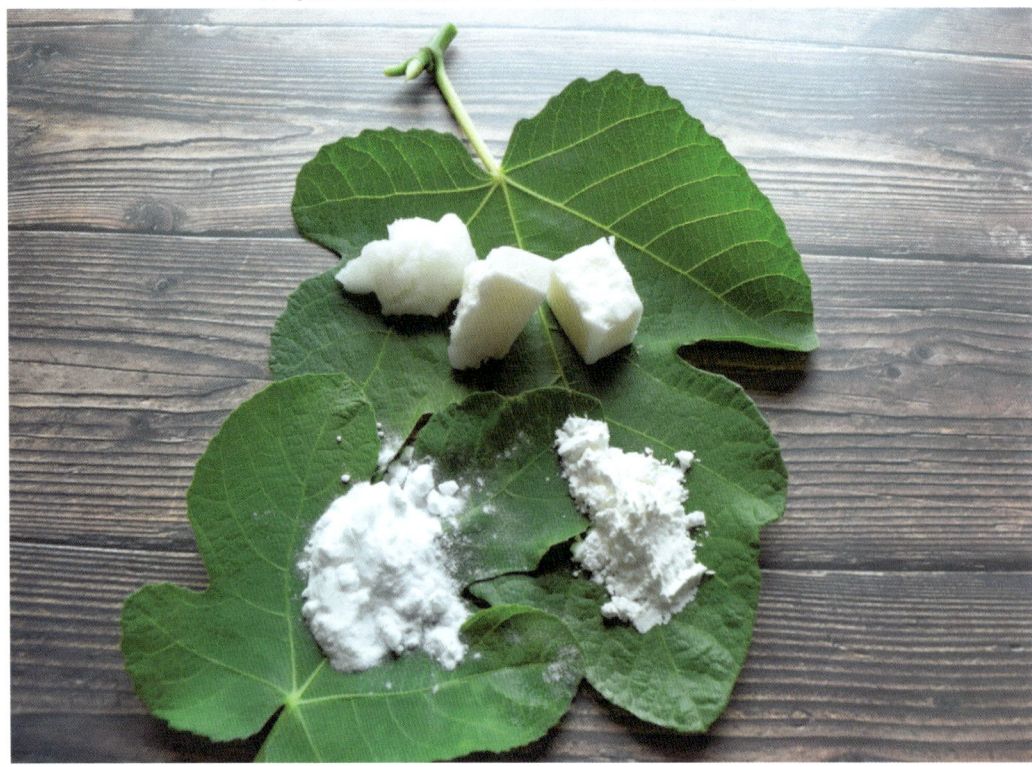

Ingredients:

2 1/2 tablespoons unrefined coconut oil
2 1/2 tablespoons unrefined shea butter
1/4 cup arrowroot
1 1/2 tablespoons baking soda
6 drops lavender essential oil
6 drops grapefruit essential oil
1 drop tea tree essential oil (optional)*
small jar with a lid

Directions: Place coconut oil and shea butter in a small glass bowl and melt on low in the microwave, stir occasionally. When it is melted, add in the arrowroot, baking soda and essential oils and mix well. Pour into a small jar and let cool until it has hardened.

How to use: Spoon out a pea-sized amount with a wooden scoop or with fingers and rub between fingers before applying directly to underarms. If you work out you may need to apply again later in the day.

Benefits: Coconut oil may be linked to some potential benefits for skin, including reducing inflammation, keeping skin moisturized and helping heal wounds. The medium-chain fatty acids found in coconut oil also possess antimicrobial properties that can help treat acne and protect the skin from harmful bacteria. Baking soda is effective at absorbing all types of moisture, including sweat, which makes it useful for keeping your underarms dry. It also effectively kills odor causing bacteria. Shea butter also has anti-inflammatory and healing properties. Using shea butter on your body can condition, tone, and soothe your skin. Tea tree and lavender are natural antibacterial agents. Arrowroot absorbs oils.

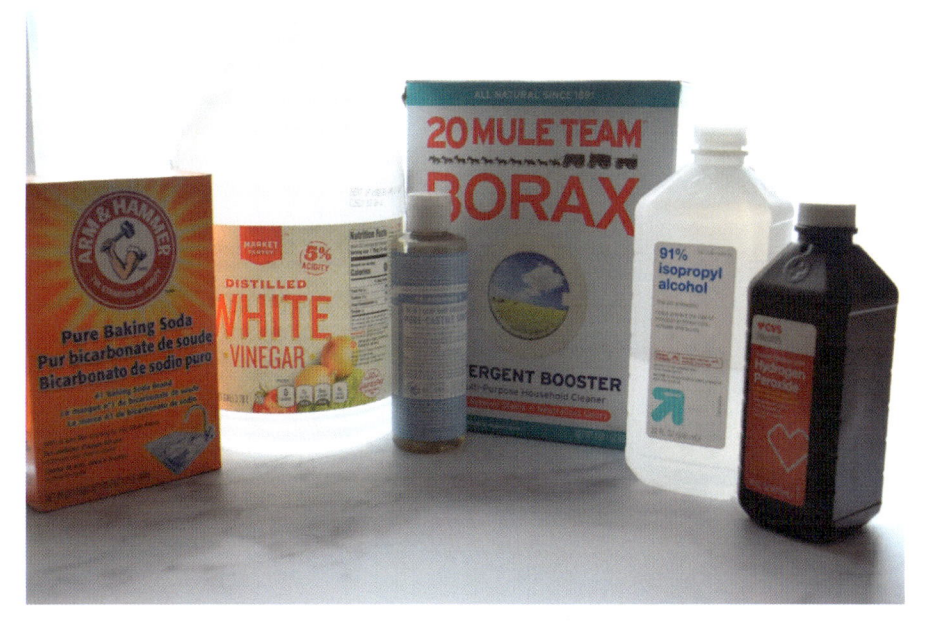

Household Cleaning Products

Free yourself from chemicals! Stock your cleaning caddy with natural cleaning agents. Baking soda works great on greasy messes and can be used as a scouring agent. It is also a natural deodorizer. Distilled white vinegar works on alkaline substances by dissolving scale, inhibiting mold and cutting soap scum. It is terrific for removing rust stains too as well as making things shiny and clean. Hydrogen peroxide is water with an extra oxygen molecule in it. It is good for an alternative to bleach. Borax is an alkali that is a great odor neutralizer and cleaner. Essential oils such as tea tree, lavender, eucalyptus and lemon enhance the scent of cleaners plus they have antibacterial properties. Castile soap is a vegetable based olive oil soap that can be used to clean a lot of things. As you can see there are many natural alternatives for household cleaners. You will learn how to make so many useful cleaning solutions in this section.

Lavender Linen Water

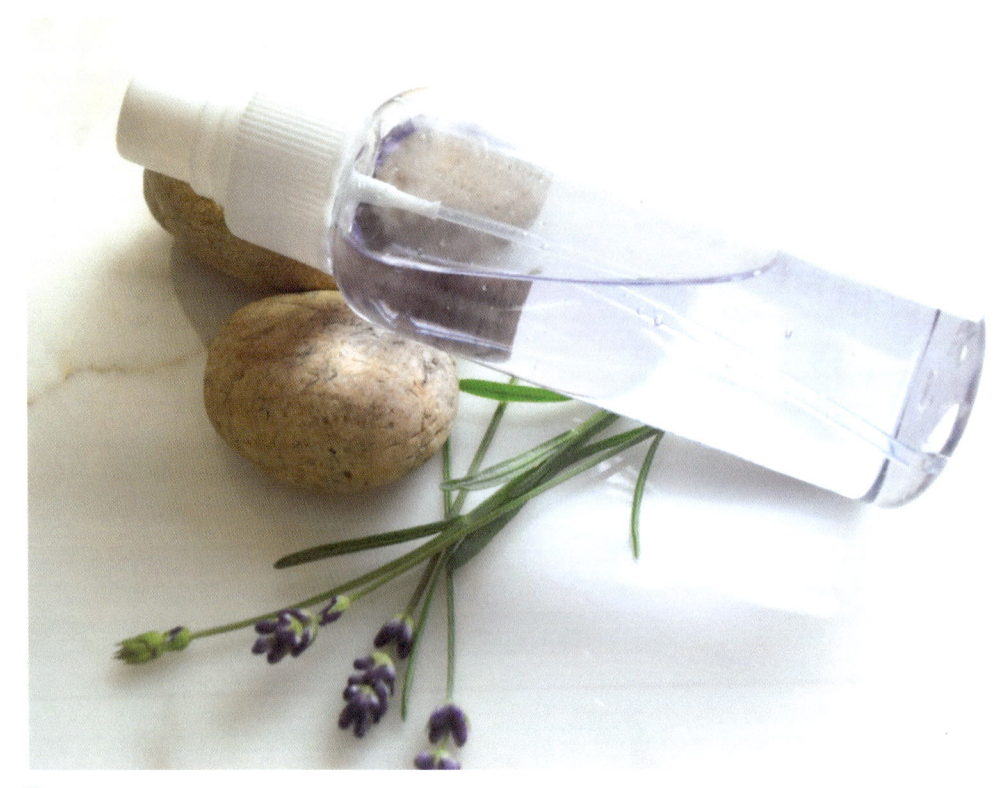

Ingredients:

4 cups of distilled water
1/2 cup of dried lavender buds
1/4 cup witch hazel
2 tablespoons of rubbing alcohol or vodka to prevent mold
25 drops lavender essential oil
spray bottle

Directions:

Add the lavender buds to the water and simmer for 15 minutes then strain. Mix all ingredients together in a spray bottle. Shake well before use.

How to use:

Spray on your linens, pillows, blankets, drapes and sofa to refresh the fabric and get rid of stale odors. You can also use this lavender linen water as a pillow spray to help you relax and sleep better.

Benefits:

Lavender has been used since ancient times to purify and cleanse. Lavender is very aromatic and herbaceous. It has a slightly sweet fragrance. The essential oil has healing properties for the skin. It is used in many bath and body products. Lavender essential oil has natural antibacterial and antidepressant properties. The fragrance is calming and relaxing. Lavender is one of the most popular essential oil used in aromatherapy. It is believed to treat anxiety, fungal infections, allergies, depression, insomnia and eczema. It is also believed to have antiseptic and anti-inflammatory properties. Aromatherapy benefits: balancing, soothing, normalizing, calming, relaxing, and healing.

Linen Spray

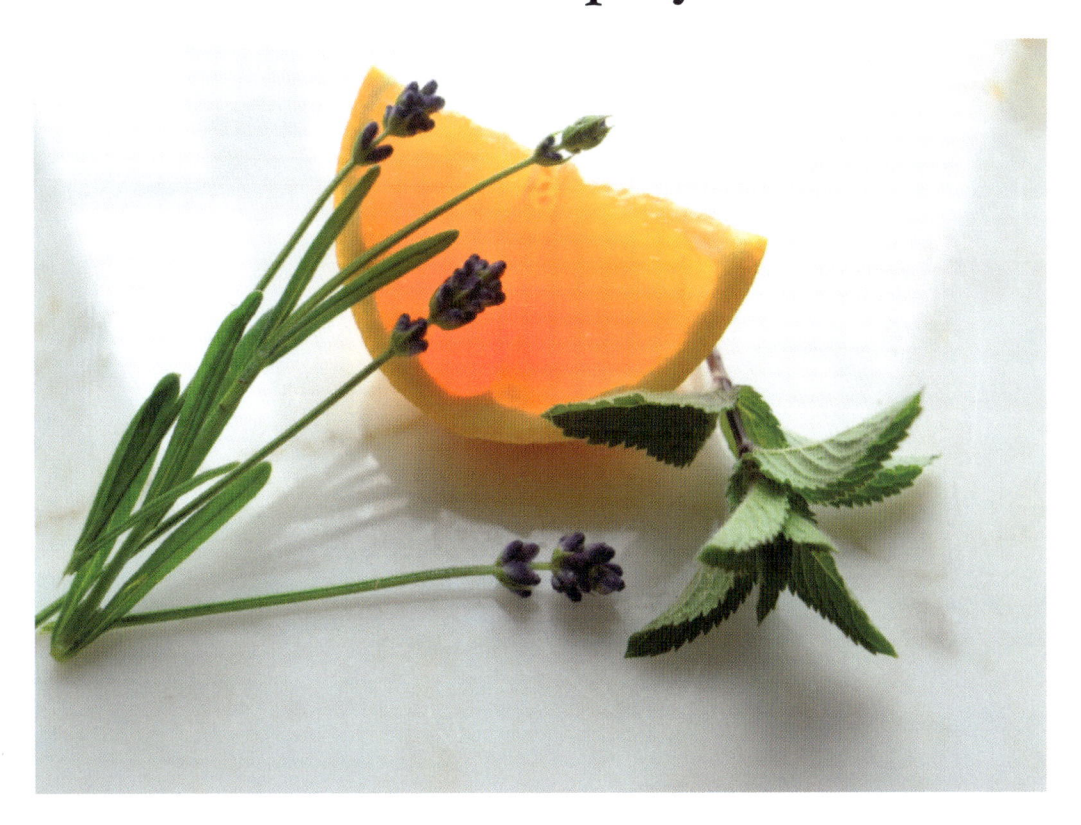

Ingredients:

1/4 cup of vodka or rubbing alcohol
1/4 cup water
20 drops of Lavender essential oil
10 drops of orange essential oil
3 drops of mint
small spray bottle

Directions: Put all ingredients in to a small spray bottle and shake gently.

How to use: Spray on your linens, pillows, blankets, drapes and sofa to refresh the fabric and get rid of stale odors.

Benefits:

Orange essential oil has a lively, fruity, and sweet aroma. The essential oil of oranges is said to be an anti-depressant because it has a cheering and refreshing fragrance. Orange essential oil is a natural anti-inflammatory, it also has anti-bacterial properties. Lavender has been used since ancient times to purify and cleanse. Lavender is very aromatic and herbaceous. It has a slightly sweet fragrance. Lavender essential oil has natural antibacterial and antidepressant properties. The fragrance is calming and relaxing. Lavender is one of the most popular essential oil used in aromatherapy. It is believed to treat anxiety, fungal infections, allergies, depression, insomnia and eczema. It is also believed to have antiseptic and anti-inflammatory properties. Aromatherapy benefits: balancing, soothing, normalizing, calming, relaxing, and healing. Mint essential oil has anti-inflammatory and astringent properties. It's vitalizing and refreshing it energizes the mind and body.

Bleach Free Surface Cleaning and Disinfecting

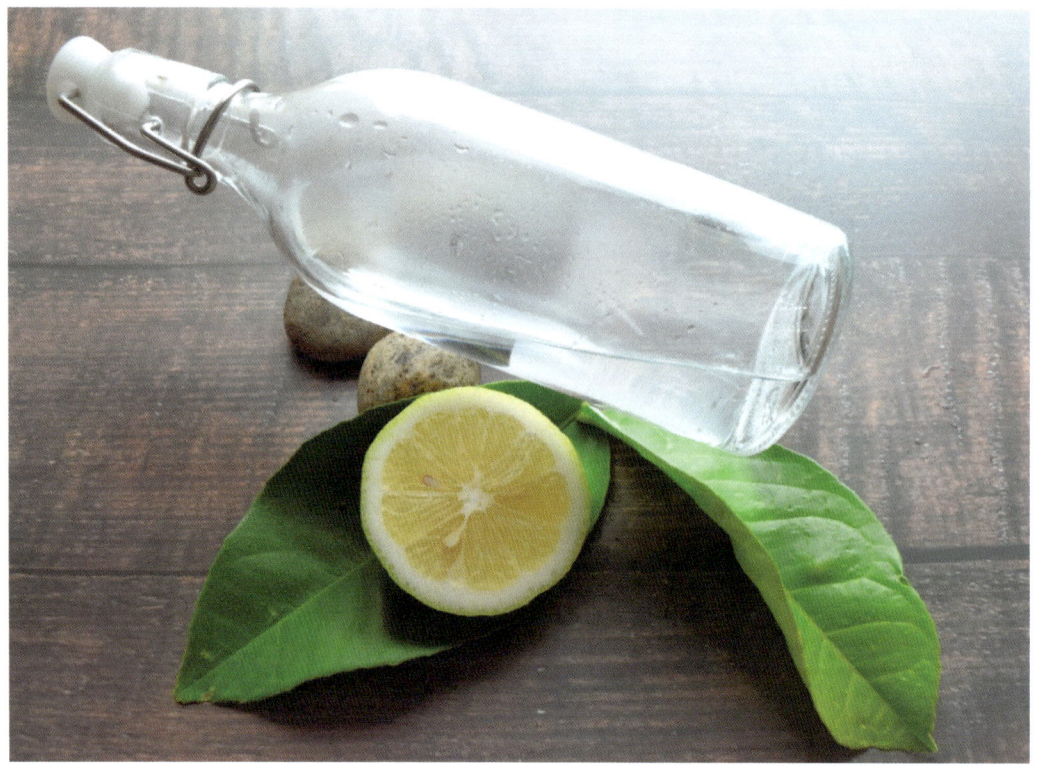

Hydrogen Peroxide & Tea Tree Oil solution # 1

Ingredients:

3 cups water,
1/4 cup hydrogen peroxide
2 tablespoons lemon juice (freshly squeezed)
10 drops Tea tree oil.
spray bottle

Tea Tree Oil & Lavender Spray solution #2

Ingredients:

16 oz spray bottle
1 ounce tea tree oil
1 ounce of Lavender essential oil.
1/4 cup of rubbing alcohol
fill the rest of the bottle with water.

Directions: Mix all ingredients together in the spray bottle. Shake before each use.

Benefits: Tea tree oil is warm, spicy, medicinal and volatile. Aromatherapy benefits: cleansing, purifying, uplifting. The oil possesses antibacterial, anti-inflammatory, antiviral, and anti-fungal properties. Lavender is very aromatic and herbaceous, slightly sweet. Lavender essential oil has natural antibacterial and antidepressant properties. Lavender oil is believed to have antiseptic properties. Rubbing alcohol kills germs and sterilizes surfaces. Hydrogen peroxide kills yeasts, fungi, bacteria, viruses, and mold spores.

Spiders and Critter Spray

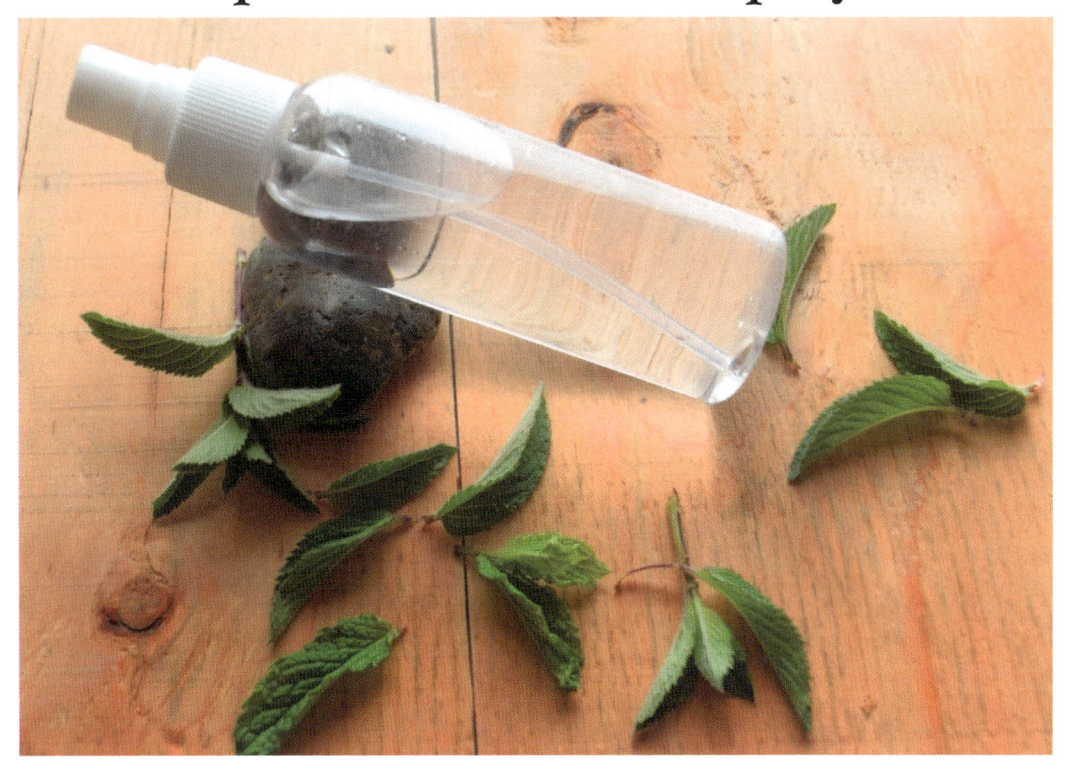

Ingredients:

30 drops of peppermint essential oil.
1 cup of water
spray bottle

Directions:

Fill a spray bottle with the water and add 30 drops of peppermint essential oil. Shake gently to mix.

How to use:

Shake before use, and then spray in the cracks and gaps where spiders and bugs can enter your home.

Benefits:

Studies have shown that this may work on mice as well. You can spray outdoors around areas where a mouse may get in. Spiders and a lot of other critters really don't like the smell of peppermint. It has a very strong scent. Peppermint essential oil is well known to help repel bugs of all sorts including ants, spiders, cockroaches, mosquitoes and mice. Peppermint has a powerful, sweet, menthol aroma which, when inhaled undiluted, can make the eyes water and the sinuses tingle.

Holiday Air Freshener

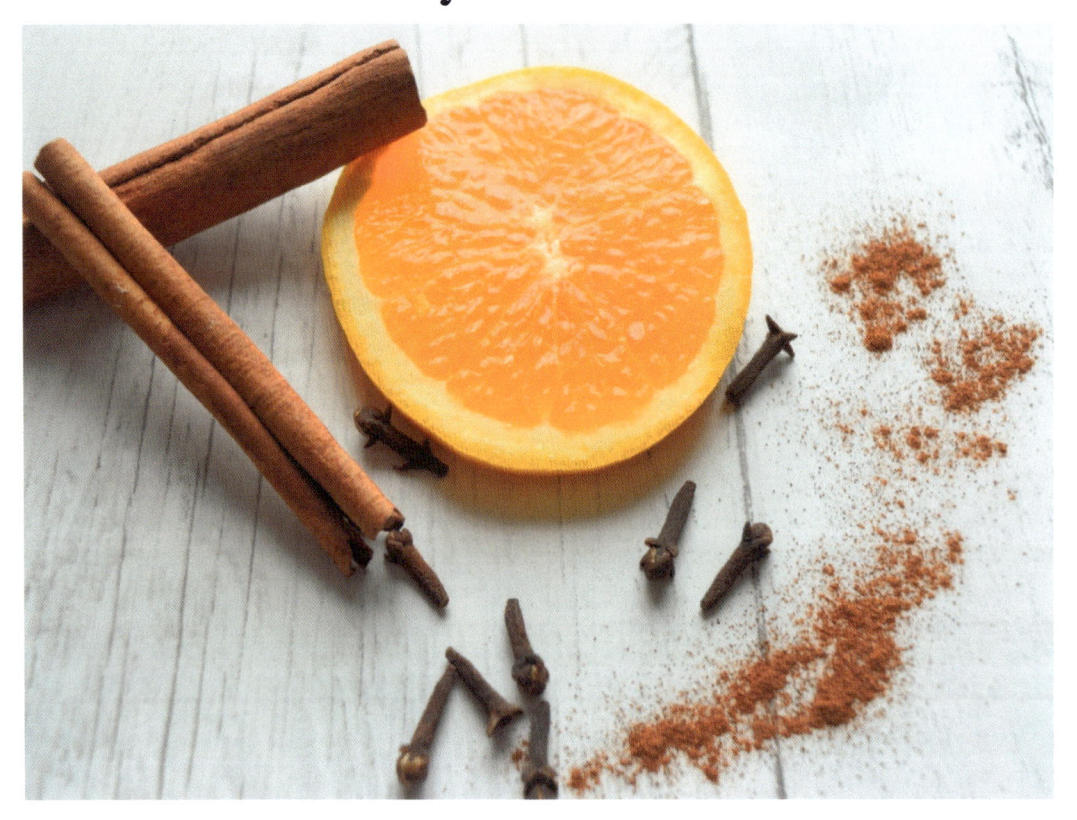

Ingredients:

4 ounces water
12 drops orange essential oil
6 drops cinnamon leaf essential oil
6 drops clove bud essential oil
spray bottle

Directions:

Place water and essential oils in spray bottle and shake to mix.

How to use:

Shake well before use and mist the air throughout your home during the holidays and all winter long.

Benefits:

Orange essential oil has a lively, fruity, sweet aroma. The essential oil of oranges is said to be an anti-depressant because it has a cheering and refreshing fragrance. Orange essential oil has anti-bacterial properties. Clove essential oil has a sweet powerful spicy fruity aroma. It is an antioxidant with natural antibiotic and antiseptic properties. Aromatherapy benefits: It is warming and comforting. Cinnamon essential oil it may help with circulation due to its warming effect and it smells good. It is stimulating and has antiseptic properties.

Air Freshener

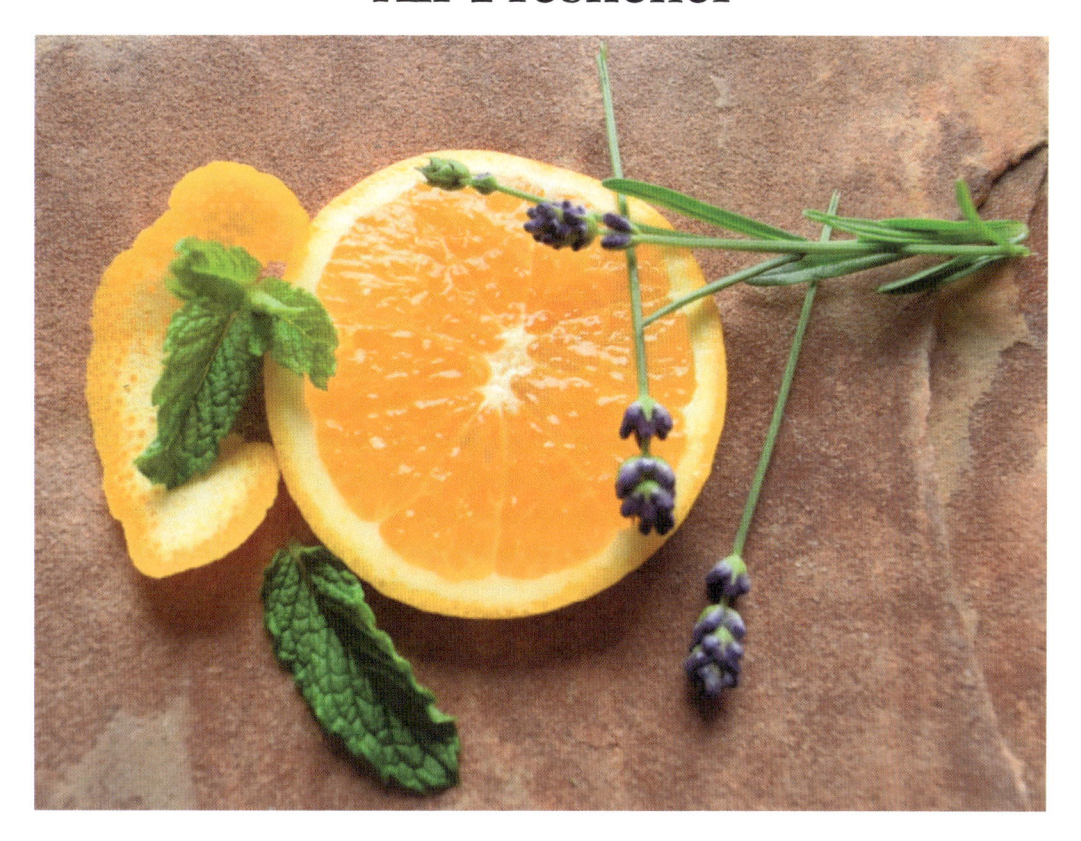

Ingredients:

3 cups water
1 cup vodka
10-20 drops of lavender essential oil
8 drops of spearmint essential oil
10 drops or orange essential oil
32 ounce spray bottle

Directions: Add all ingredients to a 32-ounce spray bottle and shake well to mix.

How to use: Shake well before use and then mist the air.

Note: Vodka is a favorite for homemade cleaners. It contains ethyl alcohol, a main ingredient in many store bought air fresheners. Any kind of vodka will work, so there's no need to buy an expensive brand.

Benefits:

Orange essential oil has a lively, fruity, sweet aroma. The essential oil of oranges is said to be an anti-depressant because it has a cheering and refreshing fragrance. Orange essential oil is a natural anti-inflammatory, it also has anti-bacterial properties. Lavender is very aromatic and herbaceous. It has a slightly sweet fragrance. Lavender essential oil has natural antibacterial and antidepressant properties. Aromatherapy benefits: balancing, soothing, normalizing, calming, relaxing, and healing. Lavender also has natural antibacterial properties. Spearmint essential oil is refreshing, cooling and vitalizing. It has a clean crisp scent. Aroma therapists use spearmint to energize the mind and body.

Natural Disinfecting Spray

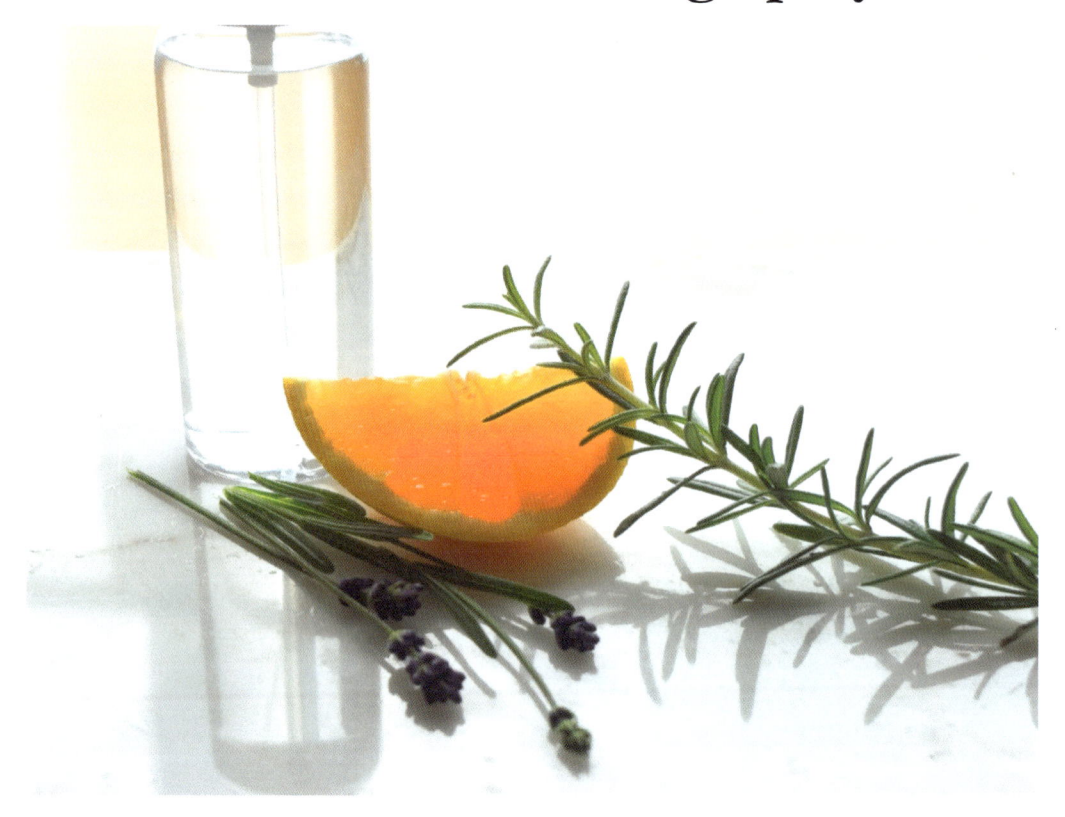

Ingredients:

1/2 cup rubbing alcohol
1/4 cup water
1/4 cup vinegar
15 drops rosemary essential oil
25 drops orange essential oil
15 drops eucalyptus essential oil
15 drops lavender oil
8-10 ounce spray bottle

Directions: Add all of the ingredients to the spray bottle and shake well.

How to use: Spray surfaces that you want to disinfect. This is best used on hard surfaces; test a small area on marble etc. before you use it.

Benefits:

Orange essential oil kills bacteria it may also prevent the growth of fungi. Eucalyptus is a germicide. Eucalyptus also has natural antibacterial properties. Lavender in a natural antiviral and antibacterial. Rosemary is a natural anti-microbial agent. Rubbing alcohol kills germs and sterilizes surfaces. Vinegar is moderately acidic, which makes it an excellent multi-purpose cleaner for house cleaning. As a household cleaner, white vinegar can be utilized to do anything from unclogging drains, to removing stains, to deodorizing, and disinfecting.

All Purpose Cleaner

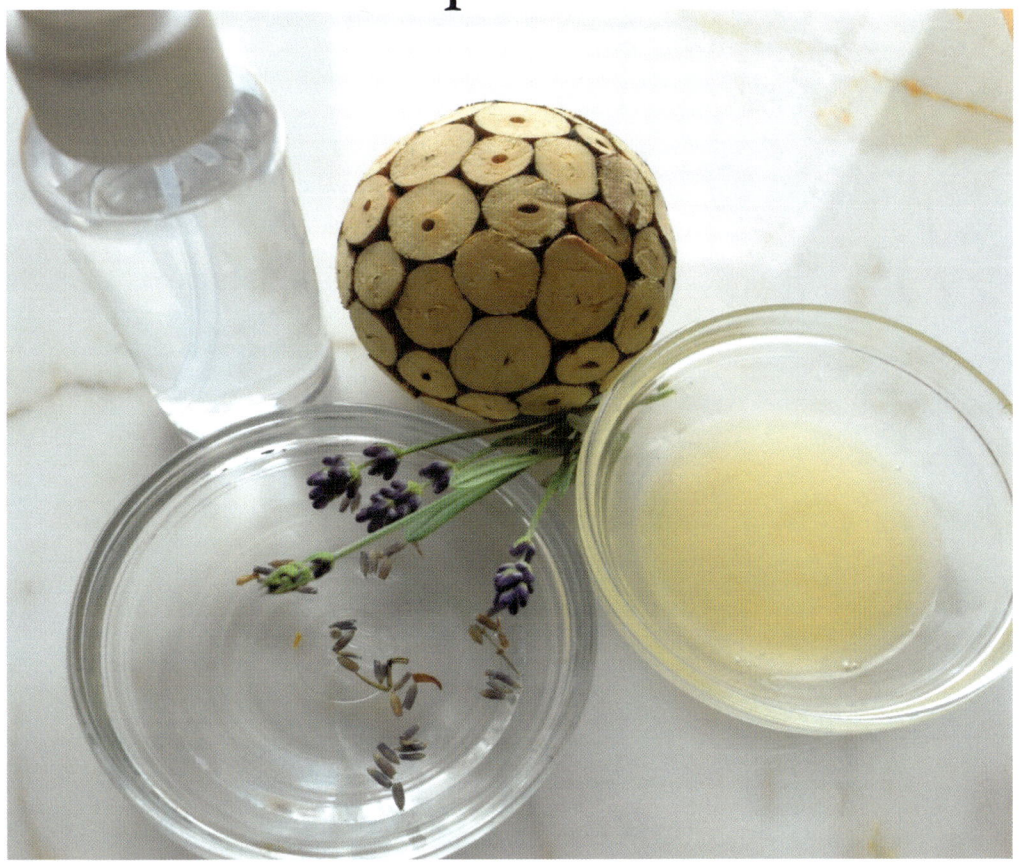

Ingredients:

3/4 cup hydrogen peroxide
1/2 cup distilled white vinegar
1 teaspoon unscented liquid Castile soap
10 drops tea tree oil
20 drops lavender essential oil
2 cups water
24 ounce spray bottle

Directions: Add all ingredients to a 24-ounce spray bottle; shake before use.

How to use: Use for general cleaning needs. For an extra boost when removing mildew and soap buildup, spray first, then sprinkle on baking soda and scrub with a sponge.

Benefits:

Hydrogen peroxide is water with an extra oxygen molecule in it. It is good for an alternative to bleach. Vinegar is moderately acidic, which makes it an excellent multi-purpose cleaner for house cleaning. As a household cleaner, white vinegar can be utilized to do anything from unclogging drains, to removing stains, to deodorizing, and disinfecting. Castile soap can clean multiple surfaces from counter tops to cook tops, hand dish washing, kitchen sinks and scrubbing away grease and grime. Named after the olive oil-based soaps originating in Castile, Spain, Castile soap can come in liquid or bar form, it is made only from vegetable oils Lavender is a natural antiviral and antibacterial agent. Tea tree oil possesses antibacterial, anti-inflammatory, antiviral, and anti-fungal properties.

Laundry Detergent #1

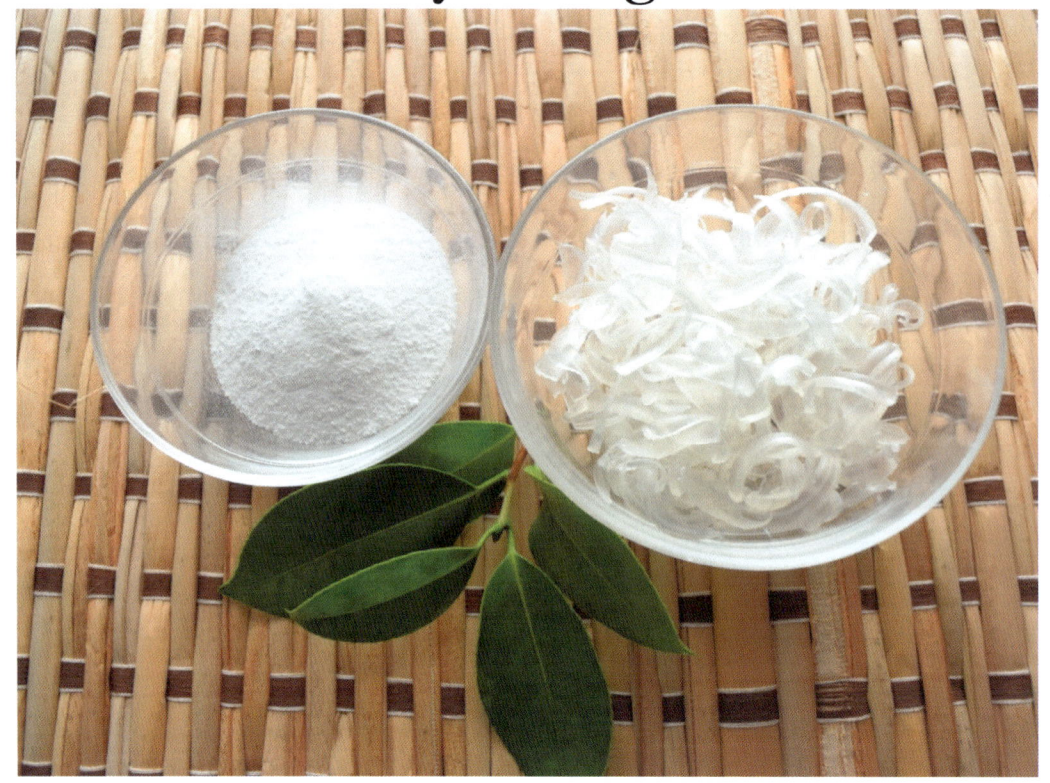

Ingredients:

1 bar laundry soap (FelsNaptha works well)
1 cup borax
1 cup washing soda (Look for it in the laundry aisle)
1 cup oxygen bleach

Directions:

Grate the bar of laundry soap; you should have about 2 cups grated soap. Mix all ingredients in a large container. Store in a container with a lid.

How to use:

Use 1/8 cup for a light load and 1/4 cup for a large or dirty load. Wash as normal.

Benefits:

Fels Naptha Soap is a fantastic stain remover and pre-treater. Borax is an alkali that is a great odor neutralizer and cleaner. It's used in laundry detergents and household cleansers to help whiten and get rid of dirt. It can neutralize odors and soften hard water. Washing soda is used to remove stubborn stains from laundry. Oxygen bleach uses a much gentler sodium percarbonate to clean laundry when mixed with water, the simple contents break down to hydrogen peroxide which is essentially water and oxygen plus sodium carbonate, or soda ash. It contains no phosphorous or nitrogen making it a perfect eco-friendly choice.

Laundry Detergent #2

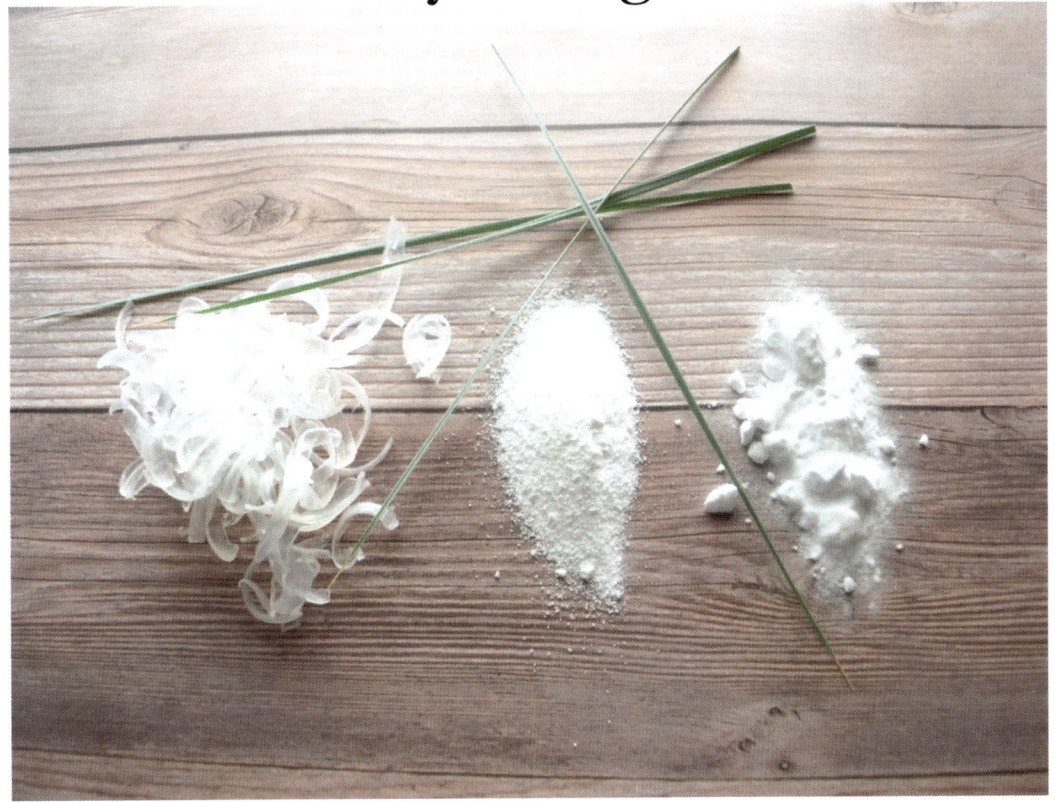

Ingredients:

2 teaspoons lavender essential oil
1 teaspoon lemon essential oil
1 teaspoon grapefruit essential oil
8 cups baking soda
6 cups borax
4 cups of grated Castile soap (about 3 to 4 bars)

Directions: Use a wire whisk to fully blend essential oils and baking soda, then whisk in the other ingredients until well combined. Use 1/8 cup for a regular-sized load. Store in an airtight container.

Benefits:

Borax is an alkali that is a great odor neutralizer and cleaner. It's used in laundry detergents and household cleansers to help whiten and get rid of dirt. It can neutralize odors and soften hard water. Castile soap can clean multiple surfaces from counter tops to cook tops, hand dish washing, kitchen sinks and scrubbing away grease and grime. Named after the olive oil-based soaps originating in Castile, Spain, Castile soap can come in liquid or bar form, it is made only from vegetable oils. Baking soda is a natural deodorizer and cleanser. Adding it to laundry is a great way to gently clean your clothes to remove tough smells and stains. Using baking soda can also help soften clothes, boost your detergent's power, and keep whites white. As a bonus, it helps your washing machine stay clean, too. The lemon, lavender and grapefruit essential oils have natural antibacterial properties plus it will make your laundry smell good.

Laundry Rinse Aid

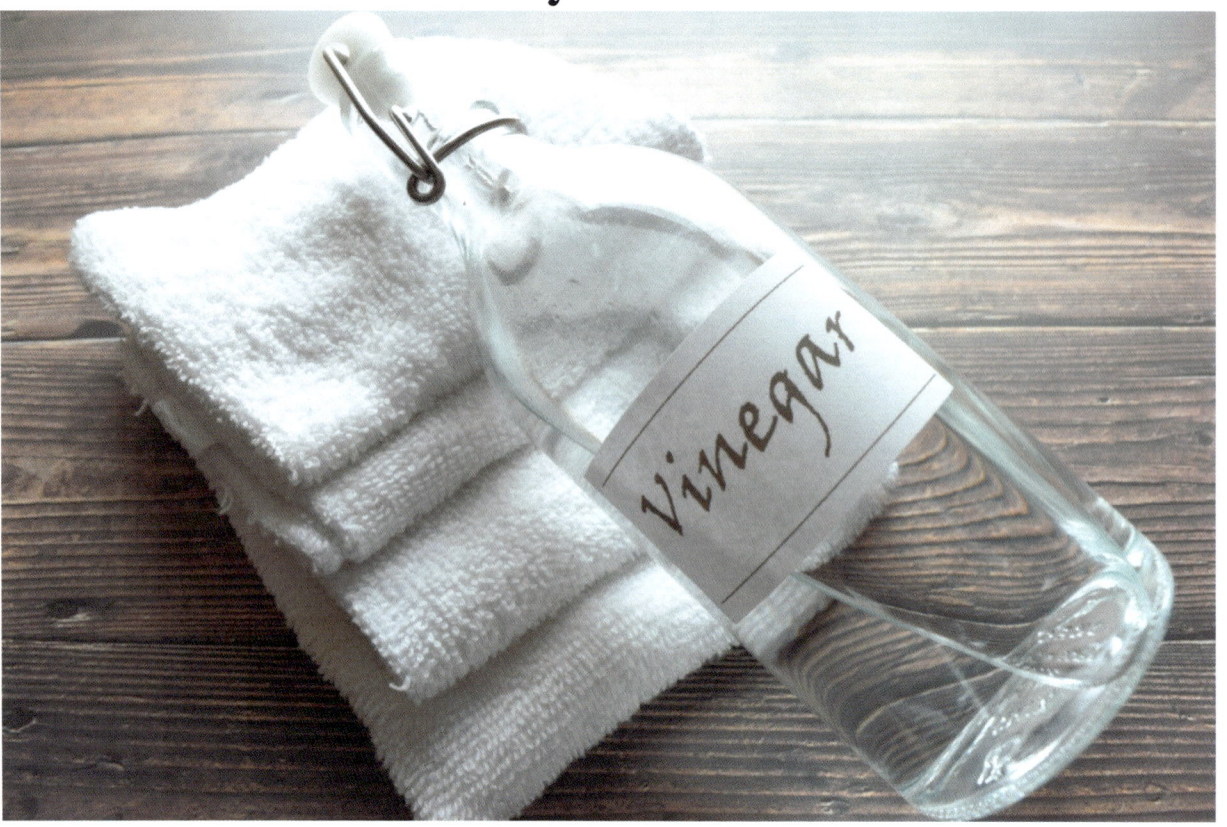

Ingredients:

1 gallon distilled white vinegar
25-30 drops essential oil of your choice

Directions:

Add the drops of essential oils to the container of vinegar and shake gently to mix.

To Use:

Use 1/4 cup in the rinse cycle.

Benefits:

Distilled white vinegar in laundry will whiten, brighten, reduce odor, and soften clothes without harsh chemicals. Vinegar is safe to use in both standard and high-efficiency washers and is beneficial to septic tanks and the environment. The essential oils will make your laundry smell good.

Window and Glass Cleaner

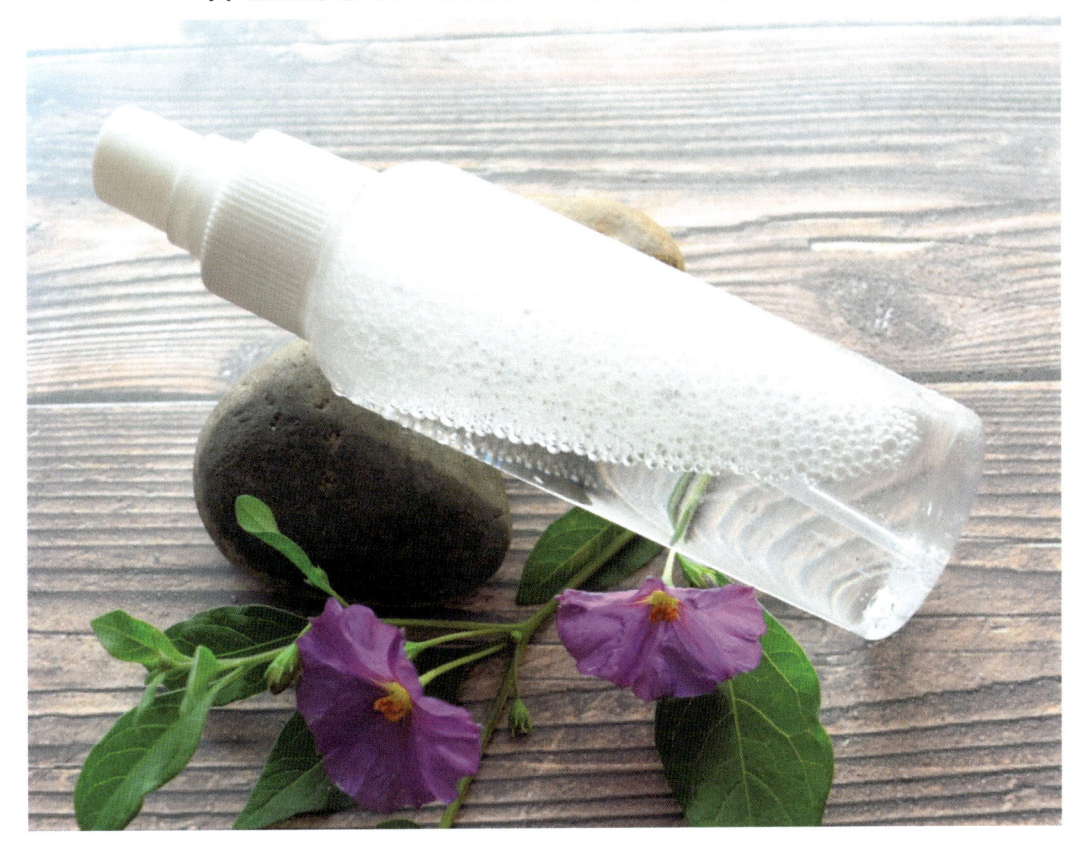

Ingredients:

2 cups water
1/4 cup distilled white vinegar
1/2 teaspoon dish soap

Directions:

Add all ingredients to a 24-ounce spray bottle. Shake to combine.

How to Use:

Use on windows, glass or fronts of appliances. Spray on and wipe off.

Benefits:

Get a streak-free sparkle with this simple cleaner, and enjoy a better view through your windows. Invest in a small stack of soft cotton or microfiber cloths for best results. Vinegar's most common and perhaps most effective cleaning application is cleaning glass, such as windows. Distilled white vinegar works on alkaline substances by dissolving scale, inhibiting mold and cutting soap scum. It is terrific for removing rust stains too as well as making things shiny and clean. The acidic nature of vinegar is so powerful it can dissolve mineral deposits, dirt, grease, and grime.

Disinfectant Wipes

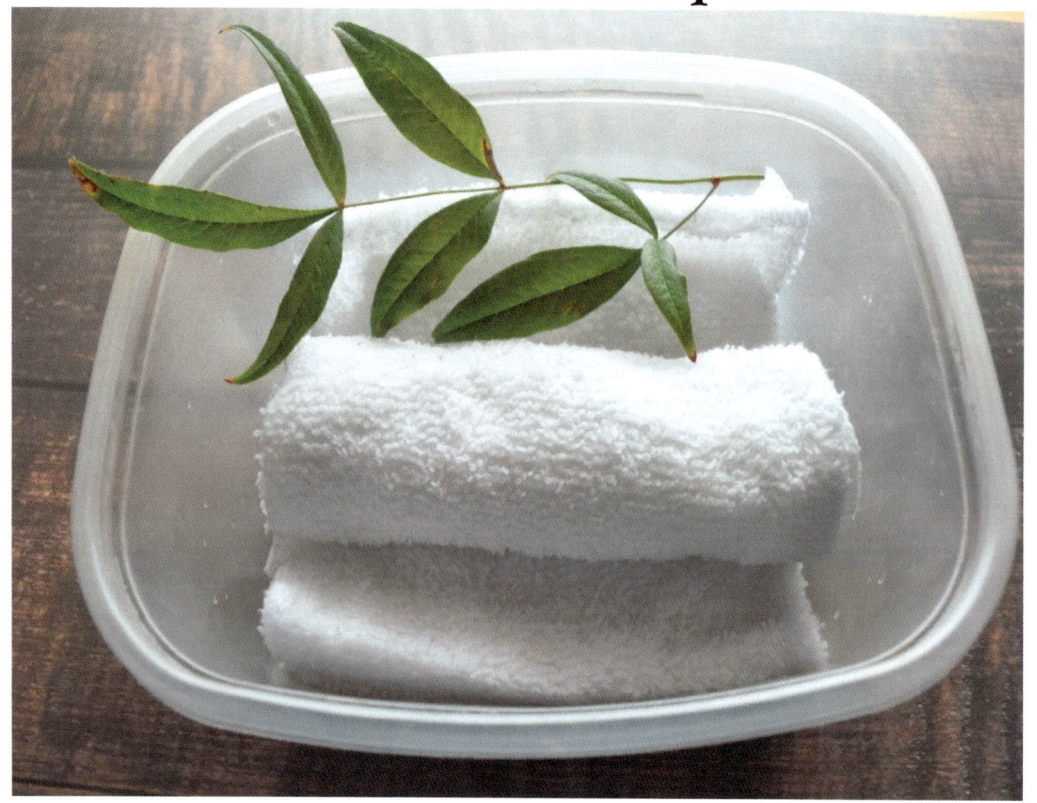

Ingredients:

1/2 cup water
1/4 cup with vinegar
1 cup rubbing alcohol
15 drops tea tree oil
10 drops eucalyptus essential oil
10 drops lemon essential oil
plastic container with a lid
10 small white wash cloths

Directions: Fold and place wash cloths into the empty plastic container and set aside. Combine in a mixing bowl the water, vinegar, alcohol and 3 essential oils, stirring until well mixed. Pour this mixture over the cloths in the container where they will soak and be ready for you to pull out and use When you are done using one just throw it in the wash. Wash in hot water.

To use: Use on counters, tables, and door knobs any where you need to clean. Do a test patch on some surfaces like marble, wood etc. before the first use.

Benefits:

The acidic nature of vinegar is so powerful it can dissolve mineral deposits, dirt, grease, and grime. It can also kill some germs. Rubbing alcohol kills germs and sterilizes surfaces. Tea tree oil possesses antibacterial, anti-inflammatory, antiviral, and anti-fungal properties. Eucalyptus oil contains substances that kill bacteria. It also may kill some viruses and fungi. Lemon essential has natural antibacterial properties.

Toilet Cleaner Tablets

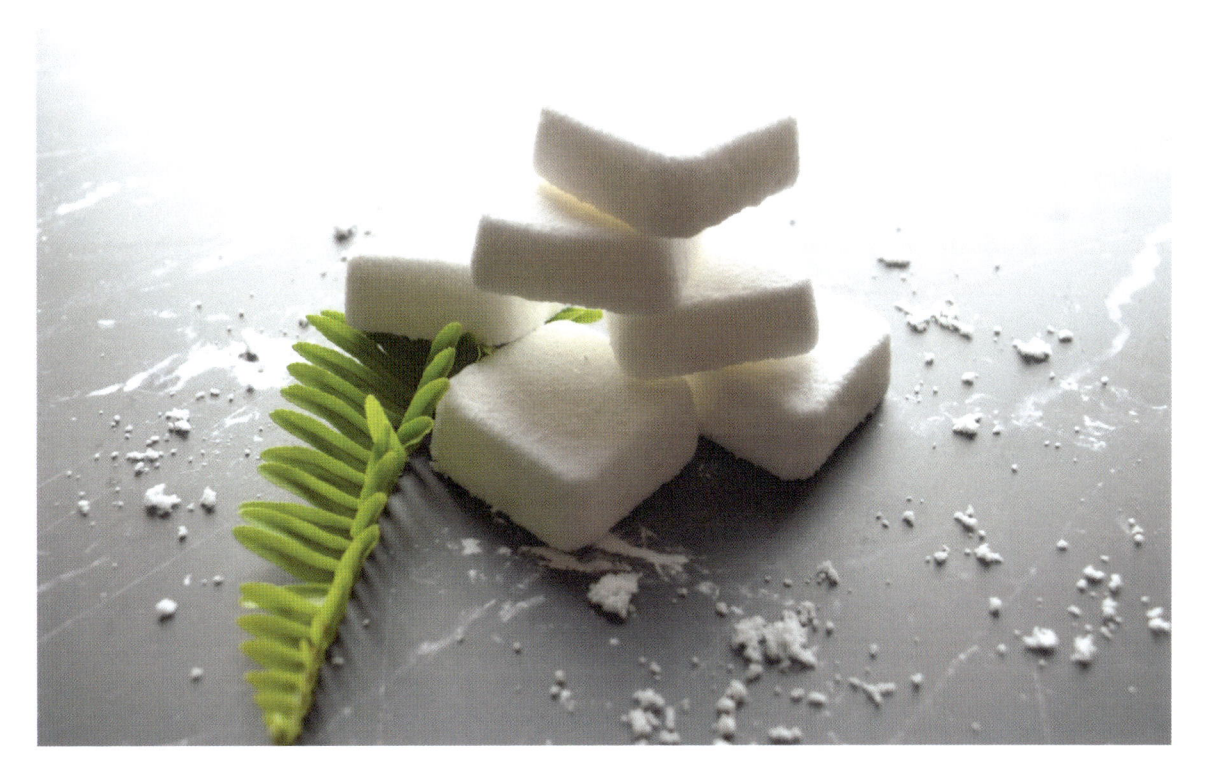

Ingredients:

1 cup baking soda
1 cup citric acid
12 drops eucalyptus essential oil
12 drops rosemary essential oil
12 drops tea tree essential oil
12 drops lemon essential oil
Silicon mold like for ice cubes

Directions:

Place all of the ingredients into a glass bowl and gently whisk together until completely blended. Scoop out and spoon into the mold and press down to compact the mixture. Let dry over night until hardened then gently pop out of the mold.

How to Use

Put 1-2 tablets into your toilet bowl and let fizz, when the fizzing stops scrub with a brush then flush the toilet.

Benefits:

The cleaning power of the baking soda and citric acid, (which causes the fizzing action) with the essential oils, will get your toilet clean. Tea tree, lemon, eucalyptus essential oils have natural antibacterial properties. No more chemicals to clean your toilet!

Wood Polishing Spray

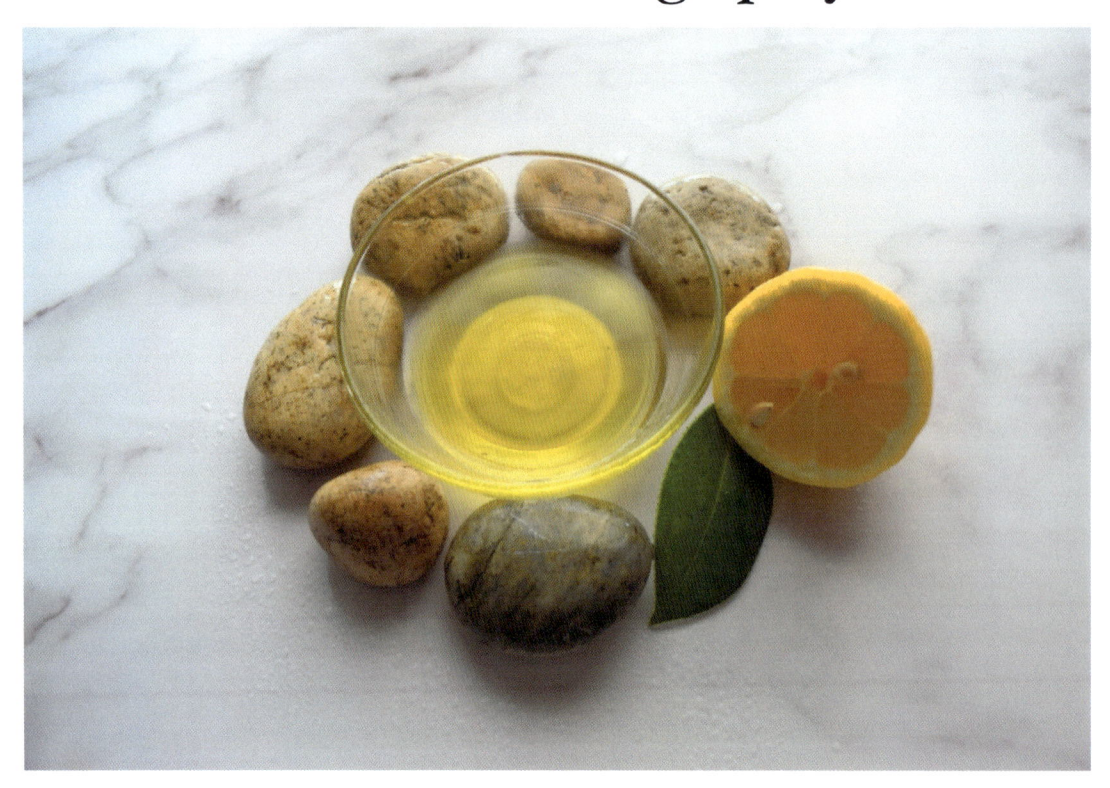

Ingredients:

3/4 cup olive oil
1/4 cup white vinegar
30 drops of lemon essential oil

Directions:

Combine ingredients in a spray bottle and shake vigorously.

How to use:

Spray directly on wood furniture and buff with a clean, dry cloth. Shake before each use.

Benefits:

Olive oil is a greener solution compared to petroleum-based wood polishes. Olive oil is eco-friendly and much cheaper to use. While some people think that the use of olive oil might damage wooden furniture, it actually nourishes the wood and brings out its natural shine. The vinegar helps to clean the wood and cut the olive oil so it won't be too oily. Lemon essential oil also nourishes wood.

Carpet Freshener

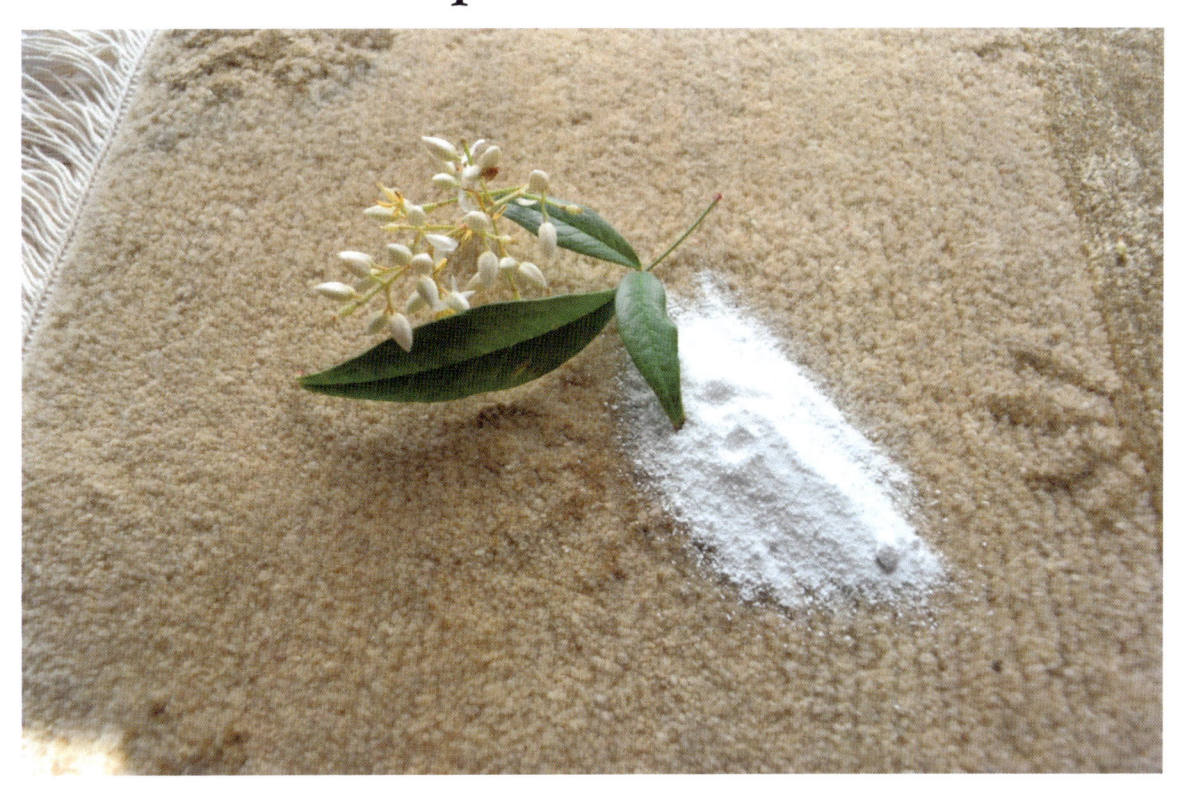

Ingredients:

2 cups borax
1 cup baking soda
10 drops essential oil of your choice

Directions:

Combine all ingredients in a bowl and mix well. Store in an air-tight container.

How to use:

Just sprinkle around the carpet and let sit for about half an hour. Vacuum up and you're done!

Benefits:

Borax is an alkali that is a great odor neutralizer and cleaner. Baking soda is also a wonderful cleaner, it absorbs oil and odors. The essential oils will make your carpet and home smell so nice.

Solution for Carpet Cleaner Machines #1

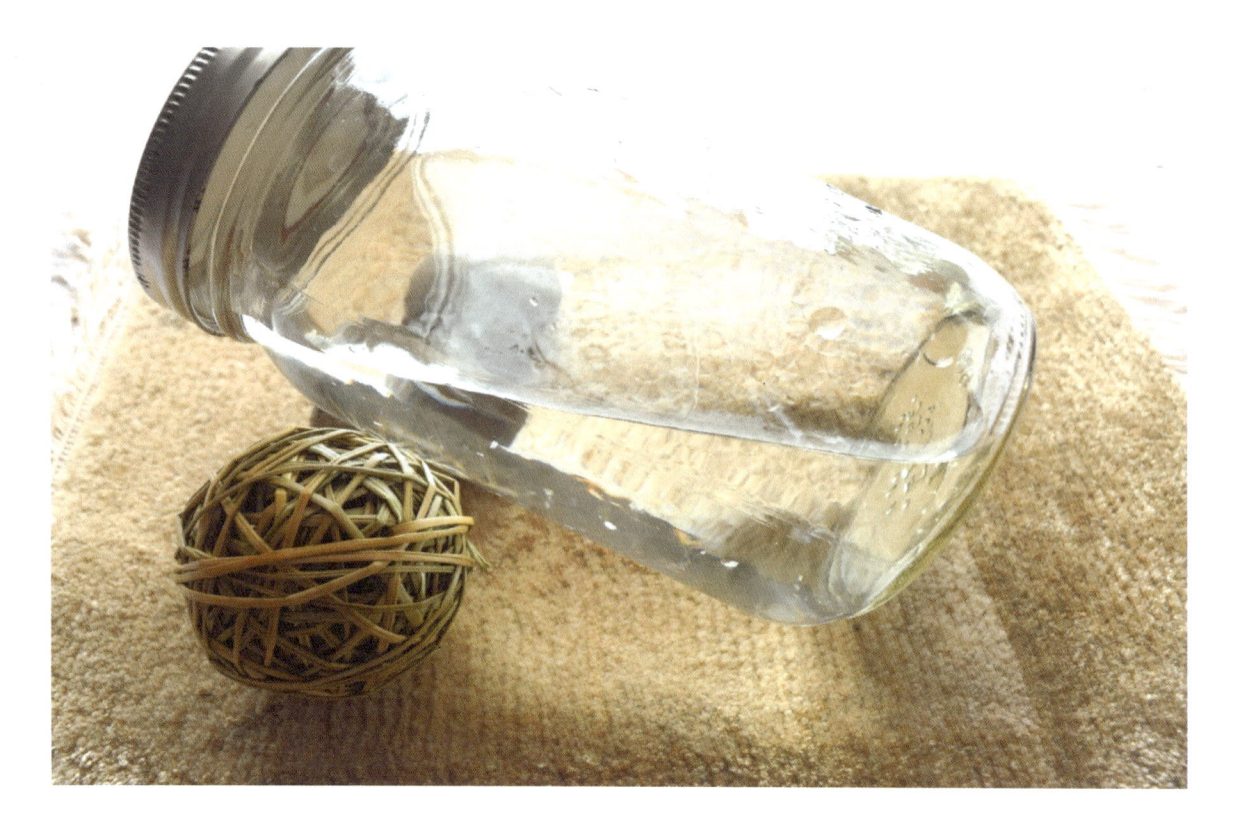

Ingredients:

1/2 gallon of white vinegar
1/2 gallon of hot water
5 drops of essential oil of your choice

Directions:

In a large bowl or pitcher combine the vinegar, hot water and essential oils mix well.

How to Use:

Before you begin to clean your carpet make sure to vacuum well. Fill the machine reservoir with the solution. Test a small patch of carpet first before doing the whole carpet to make sure it won't harm the color of your carpet. Then continue to clean the entire carpet. It should take about 8 hours to completely dry.

Benefits:

This is a basic solution that can be used regularly. It will not leave a residue on your carpet like commercial cleaners do. The vinegar is a wonderful cleaning agent that will refresh your carpet as well. Vinegar will make your carpet softer. Distilled white vinegar works on alkaline substances by dissolving scale, inhibiting mold and cutting soap scum. The acidic nature of vinegar is so powerful it can dissolve mineral deposits, dirt, grease, and grime.

Solution for Carpet Cleaner Machines #2

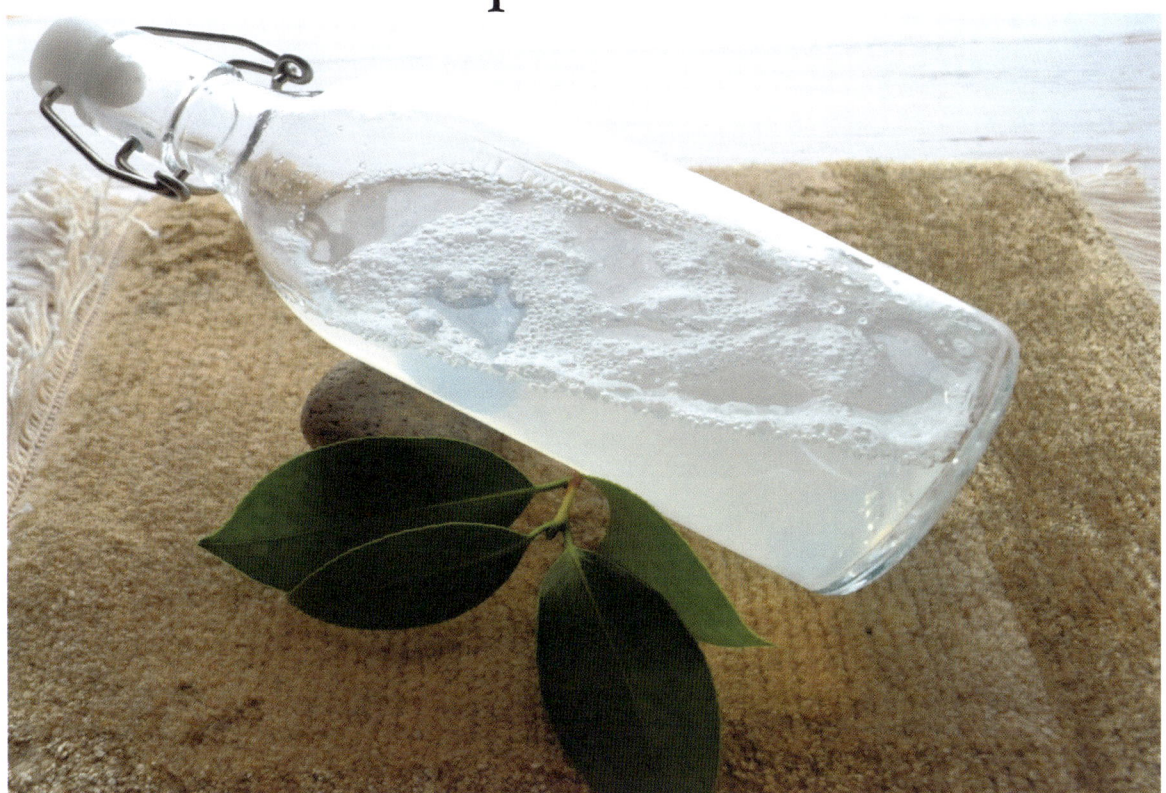

Ingredients:

1 gallon of hot water
2 tablespoons of liquid castile soap
2 tablespoons of white vinegar
2 tablespoons hydrogen peroxide
15 drops of your favorite essential oil

Directions: Combine all the ingredients in a large bowl or pitcher and mix well.

How to use:

Before you begin to clean your carpet make sure to vacuum well. Fill the machine reservoir with the solution. Test a small patch of carpet first before doing the whole carpet to make sure it won't harm the color of your carpet. Then continue to clean the entire carpet. It should take about 8 hours to completely dry.

Benefits:

Castile soap can clean multiple surfaces from counter tops to cook tops, hand dish washing, laundry, kitchen sinks and scrubbing away grease and grime. Named after the olive oil-based soaps originating in Castile, Spain, Castile soap can come in liquid or bar form, it is made only from vegetable oils. Distilled white vinegar works on alkaline substances by dissolving scale, inhibiting mold and cutting soap scum. The acidic nature of vinegar is so powerful it can dissolve mineral deposits, dirt, grease, and grime. It can make your carpets soft. Hydrogen peroxide is water with an extra oxygen molecule in it. It is good for an alternative to bleach.

Natural Floor Cleaning Solution

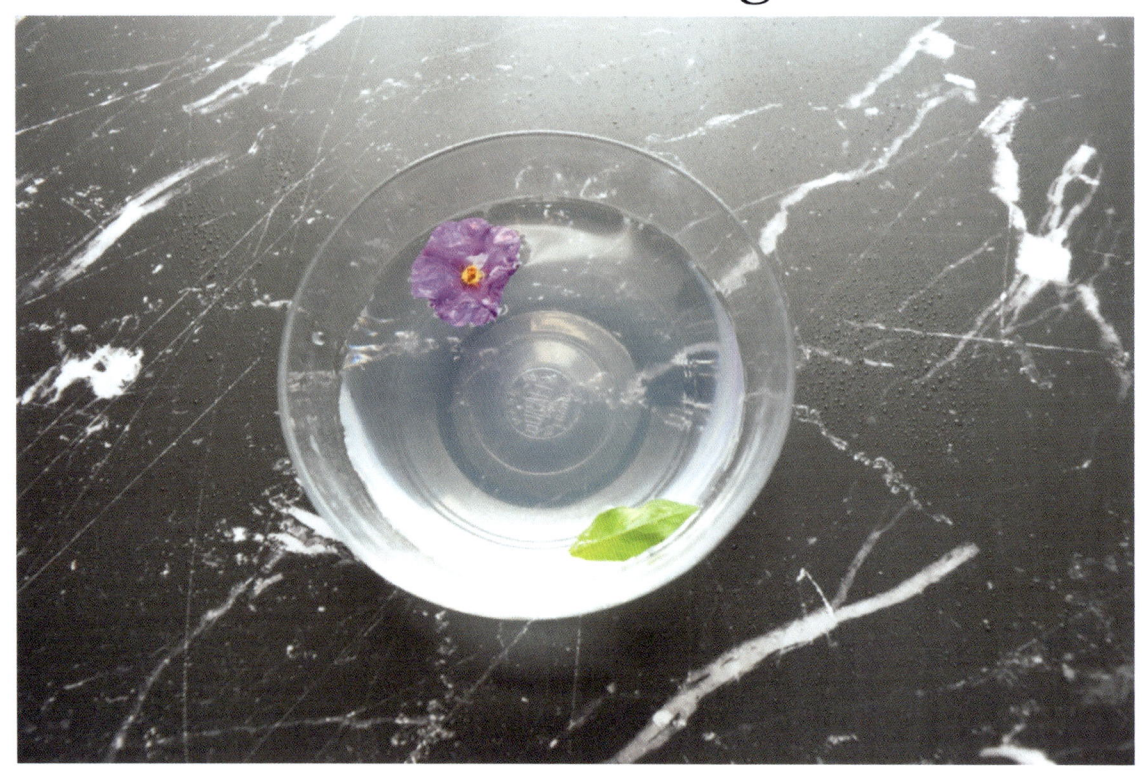

Ingredients:

1 gallon of warm water
1 cup of vinegar
1/2 cup of alcohol
1/2 teaspoon of dish soap
10-20 drops of essential oil
bucket

Directions: Fill your bucket with all of the ingredients and mix well, put your mop in the bucket and wring out and mop as usual. As always do a test patch first before using.

Notes: Do not use a liquid dish detergent that contains moisturizing, anti-bacterial, or oxygenated bleach ingredients. Also, do not swap Castile soap for the dish detergent since it is an oil-based soap and will leave streaks and make the floor slippery.

Benefits: Distilled white vinegar works on alkaline substances by dissolving scale, inhibiting mold and cutting soap scum. It is terrific for removing rust stains too as well as making things shiny and clean the acidic nature of vinegar is so powerful it can dissolve mineral deposits, dirt, grease, and grime. Rubbing alcohol kills germs and sterilizes surfaces.

Wood Cutting Board Cleaner

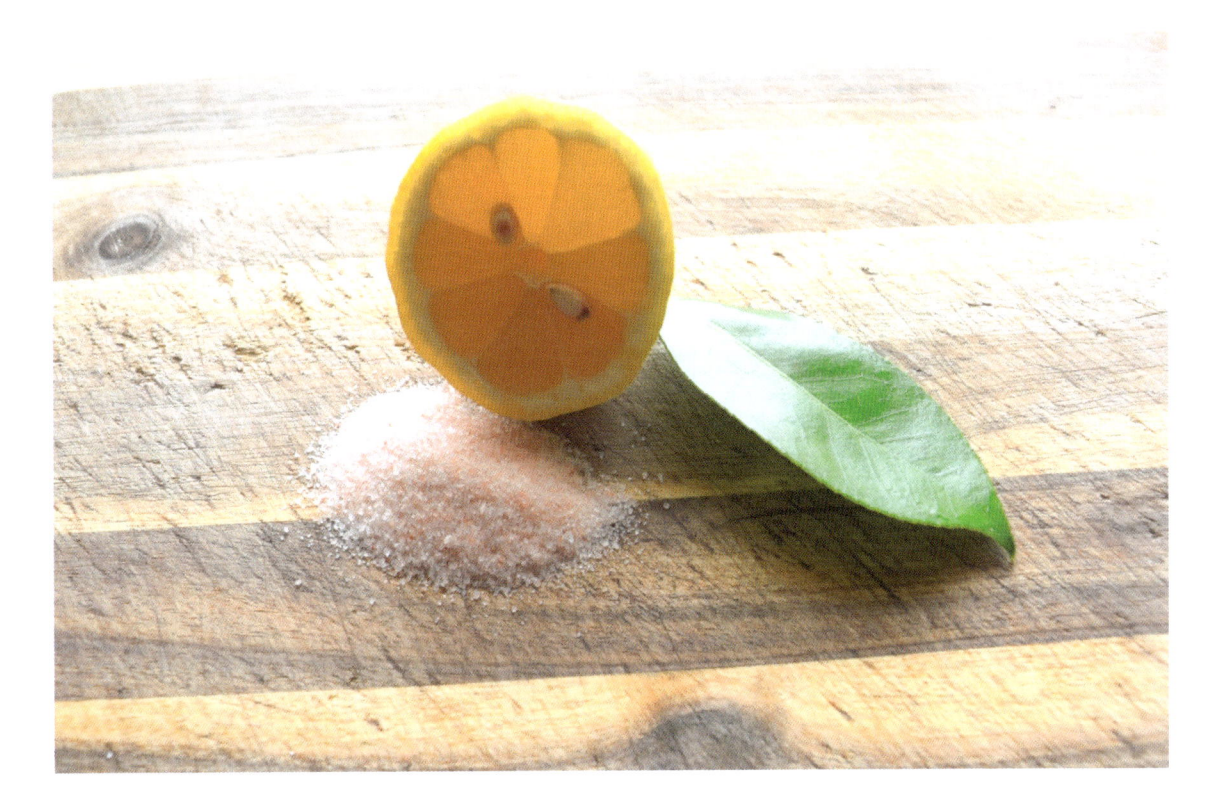

Ingredients:

1/4 cup salt
12 drops of orange essential oil.

Directions: Combine the orange essential oil with the salt.

How to use: Rub on cutting boards and rinse with hot water.

OR you can use this

Ingredients:

1/2 of a cut lemon
1/4 cup of salt

How to use: Rub the lemon in the salt then scrub your cutting board with the lemon.

Benefits: Lemon and orange essential oil both have natural antibacterial properties as well as acid that can clean. The salt also works as a scrubbing agent and can kill some bacteria.

Natural Weed Killer

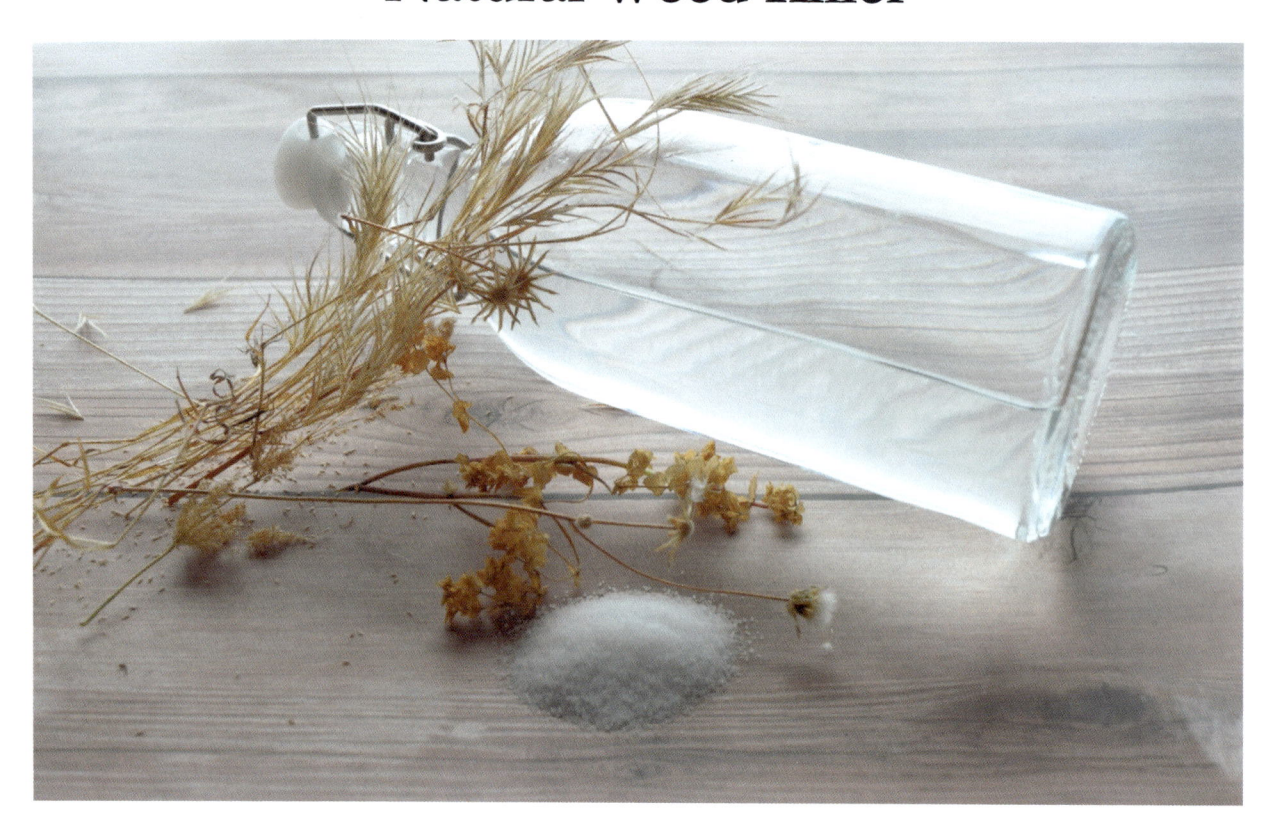

Ingredients:

1 gallon of 30% acidity vinegar
1/8 cup of salt
1/2 cup of hot water
1 garden pump sprayer

Directions:

Add the salt to the hot water and dissolve completely. The salt must be completely dissolved before you pour it into the pump sprayer. Use a little more water if you need to. Pour into the pump sprayer then add the vinegar and shake gently.

How to use:

You will need gloves, goggles and a face mask because the vinegar can burn you because of the high acid content. Also wear protective clothes. Spray the weeds during the day. The next day the weeds will be dead. Be careful where you spray you don't want the spray to get on any plants. DO NOT spray if it is windy outside. If it is raining the weed killer will not work. You have to spray on a dry wind free day.

Benefits: NO chemicals! Vinegar is all natural and this works really well. I have been using it for years. The combination of vinegar and salt dries up the weeds. Be sure to keep your pets away from the yard until the solution dries.

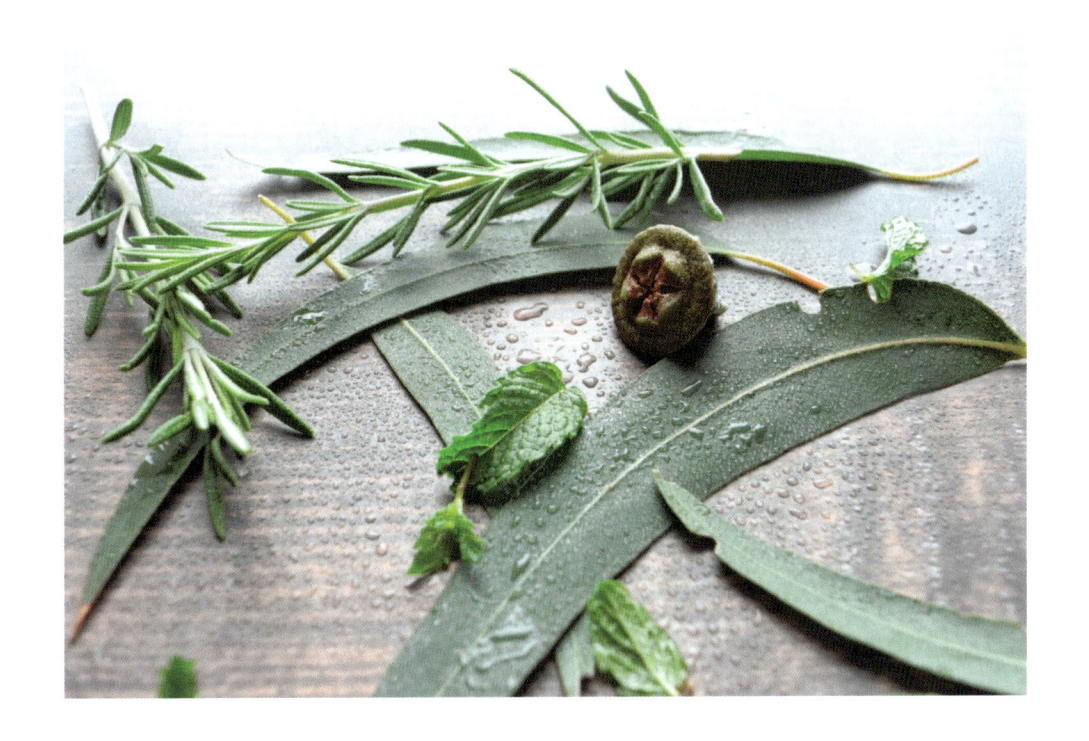

Health Products

This section is full of wonderful chemical free health products that you can make for yourself. There is Fire Cider to boost your immune system and some wonderful vapor rub to help clear up your sinuses when you have a cold. Ever wanted to make your own baby powder? There is a recipe in this section that shows you how to do that. There are recipes for Golden Milk and teas and even Elderberry syrup all of which are very healthy for your body. You may already have many of the ingredients right in your own kitchen.

Calendula Ointment

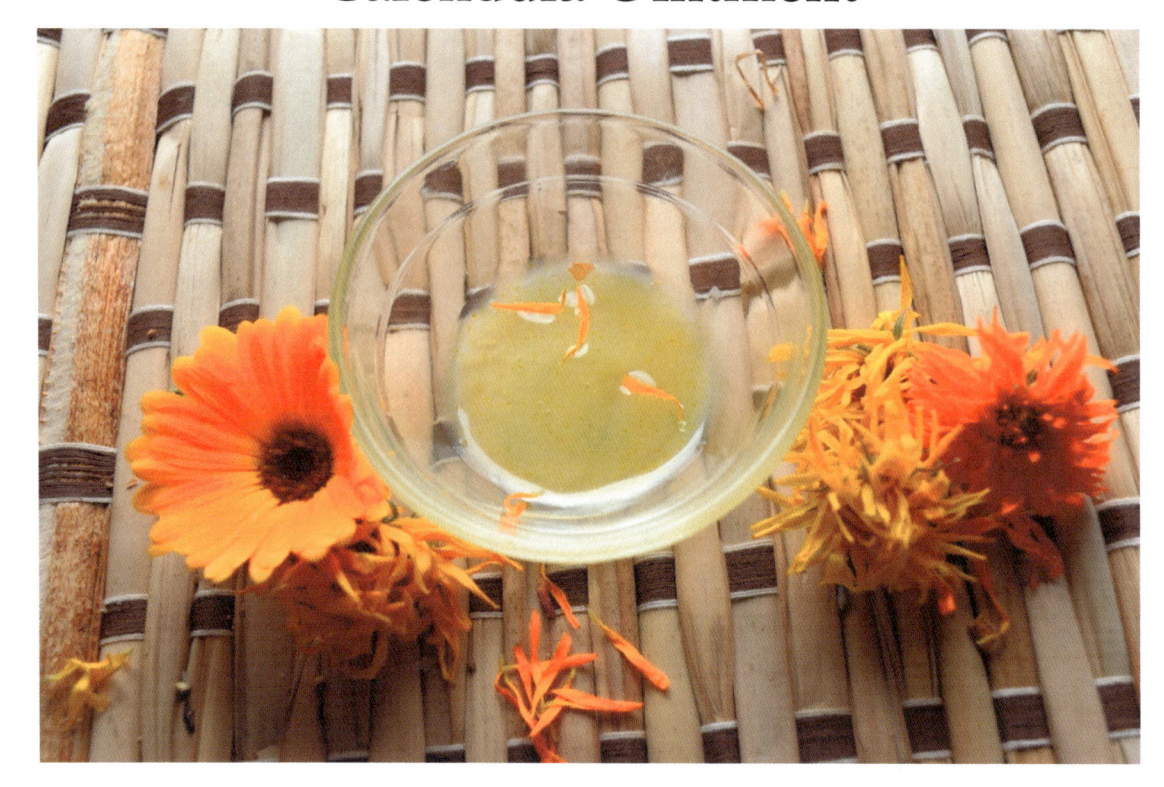

Ingredients:

1 oz. of olive oil
1 oz. of sweet almond oil
 infused with Calendula petals*
3 oz. coconut oil
1 oz. beeswax
1/2 oz. mango butter

1/2 oz. shea butter
15 drops chamomile essential oil
30 drops lavender essential oil
30 drops tea tree essential oil
1 teaspoon vitamin E
small jar with a lid

Directions: In a small glass bowl combine the butters and oils and heat gently on low in the microwave until the butters melt. Stir in the essential oils then pour into a container.

*To make infused oil: Fill a glass jar 2/3 of the way full with dried Calendula flowers. Pour oil into the jar, making sure to cover the flowers by at least one inch with oil so they will have space to expand. Stir well and cap the jar tightly. Place the jar in a warm, sunny windowsill and shake once or more daily. After 4 to 6 weeks, strain the herbs out using cheesecloth. Pour the infused oil into a glass bottle and store in a cool, dark place.

Benefits: This healing ointment is full of nourishing ingredients and can help heal skin irritations. The ancient Romans were among the first to use Calendula. They used it in their food and for medicinal purposes. Calendula usually blooms around the first of every month hence the name which in Latin is diminutive of calendae, meaning "little calendar". In the Civil War the flowers were used as a healing medicine to help heal wounds. Calendula has anti-fungal, anti-inflammatory and antibacterial properties that help heal wounds, and sooth dry skin. Coconut oil, mango oil and shea butter are healing and soothing. The Lavender and Tea Tree essential oil have natural antibacterial properties.

Calendula Salve

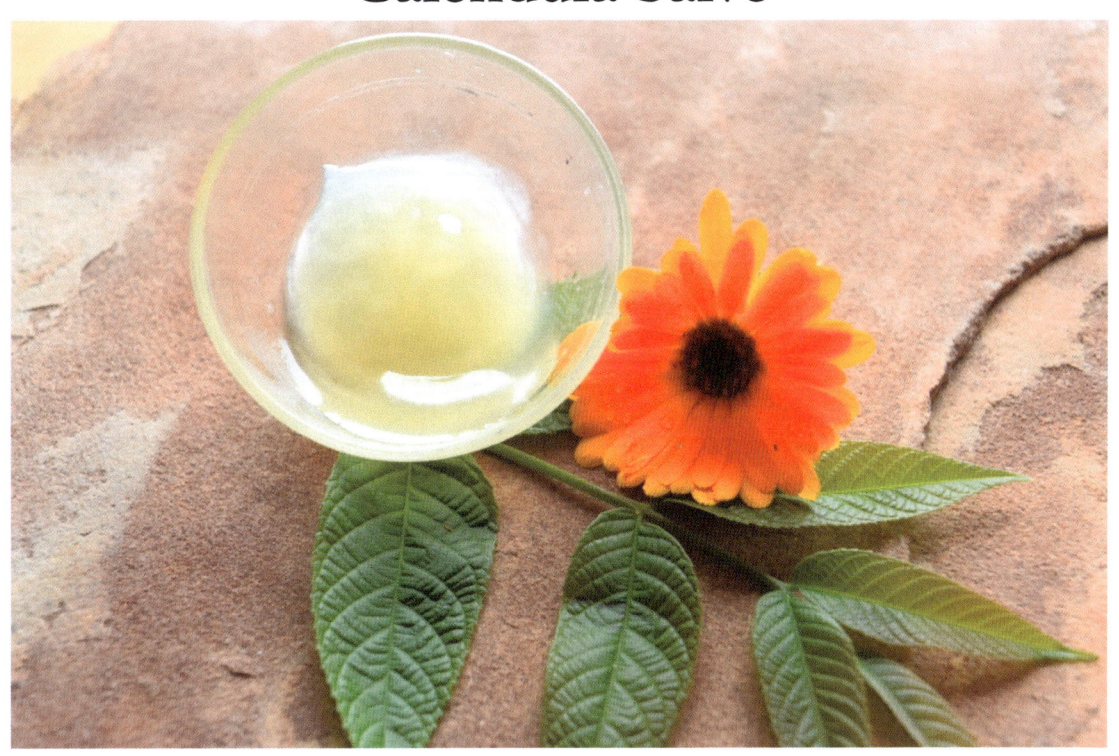

Ingredients:

4 oz. homemade Calendula-infused oil*
1/2 oz. coarsely chopped beeswax or pellets
20 drops lavender essential oil
small jar with a lid

Directions: Combine beeswax and Calendula oil in a small glass bowl and heat on low in the microwave until beeswax has melted. Mix well. Stir in lavender essential oil. Pour into a glass jar. Allow salve to cool completely before placing lid on the container. Store in a cool, dry place. If stored properly, salves can last 2 to 3 years.

How to use: To ease minor skin conditions such a bruises, small cuts or dry chapped skin, just rub a small amount into the affected area.

*To make infused oil: Fill a glass jar 2/3 of the way full with dried Calendula flowers. Pour any oil you like into the jar, making sure to cover the flowers by at least one inch with oil so they will have space to expand. Stir well and cap the jar tightly. Place the jar in a warm, sunny windowsill and shake once or more daily. After 4 to 6 weeks, strain the herbs out using cheesccloth. Pour the infused oil into a glass bottle and store in a cool, dark place.

Benefits:

The ancient Romans were among the first to use Calendula. They used it in their food and for medicinal purposes. Calendula usually blooms around the first of every month hence the name which in Latin is diminutive of calendae, meaning "little calendar". In the Civil War the flowers were used as a healing medicine to help heal wounds. Calendula has anti-fungal, anti-inflammatory and antibacterial properties that help heal wounds, and sooth dry skin.

Vapor Rub

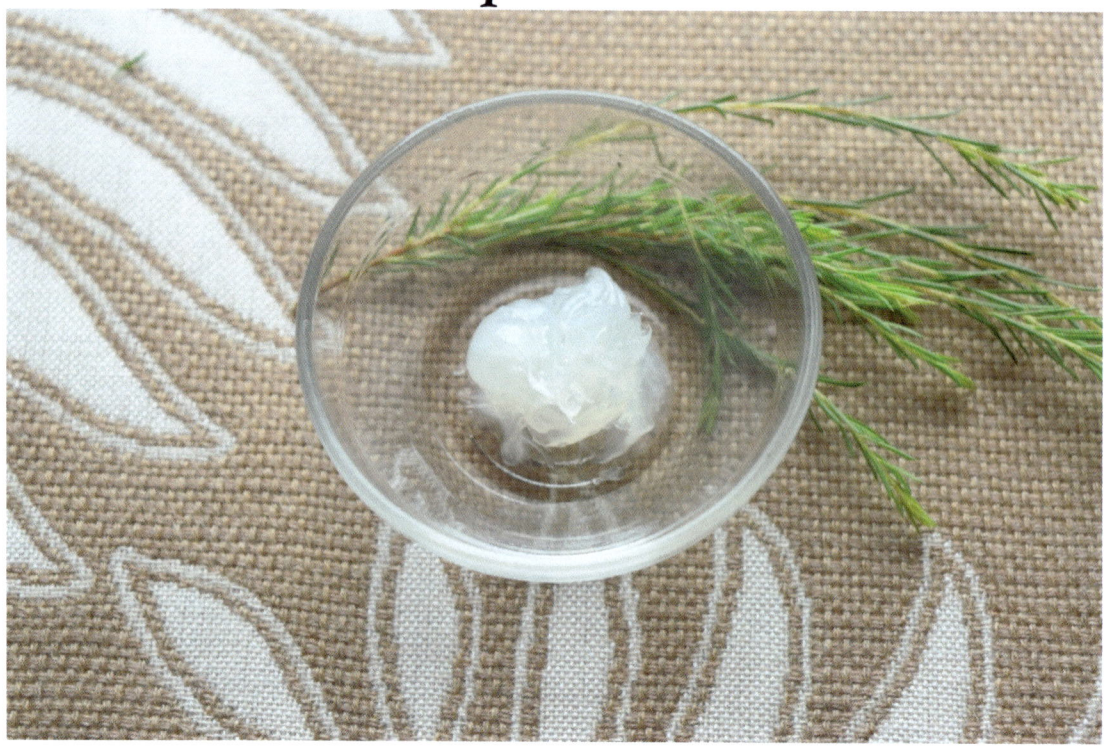

Ingredients:

1/4 cup olive oil
2 teaspoons bees wax
25-30 drops of eucalyptus essential oil
20-25 drops rosemary essential oil
10-15 drops peppermint essential oil
small glass jar with a lid

Directions:

Melt the olive oil and beeswax in a small double boiler on low heat until melted. Stir to mix well. Turn off the heat and stir in the essential oils drop by drop (keep stirring until all have been added). Pour into a small glass jar and let cool completely before putting the lid on. Store in a cool, dry place for up to a year.

How to use: Rub onto the chest and back, this should help stuffy noses and ease breathing.

Benefits:

Eucalyptus has long been used in topical preparations such as liniments and salves. It has antibacterial, anti-fungal and antiseptic properties. It works to open the sinuses. Rosemary is an ancient herb that has been used for thousands for years. The essential oil has a strong pungent scent with a hint of pine. It can help circulation and is a natural antioxidant. It is very invigorating. Peppermint essential oil has anti-inflammatory and astringent properties. Peppermint oil can be used to clear your sinuses and reduce congestion.

Detox Bath

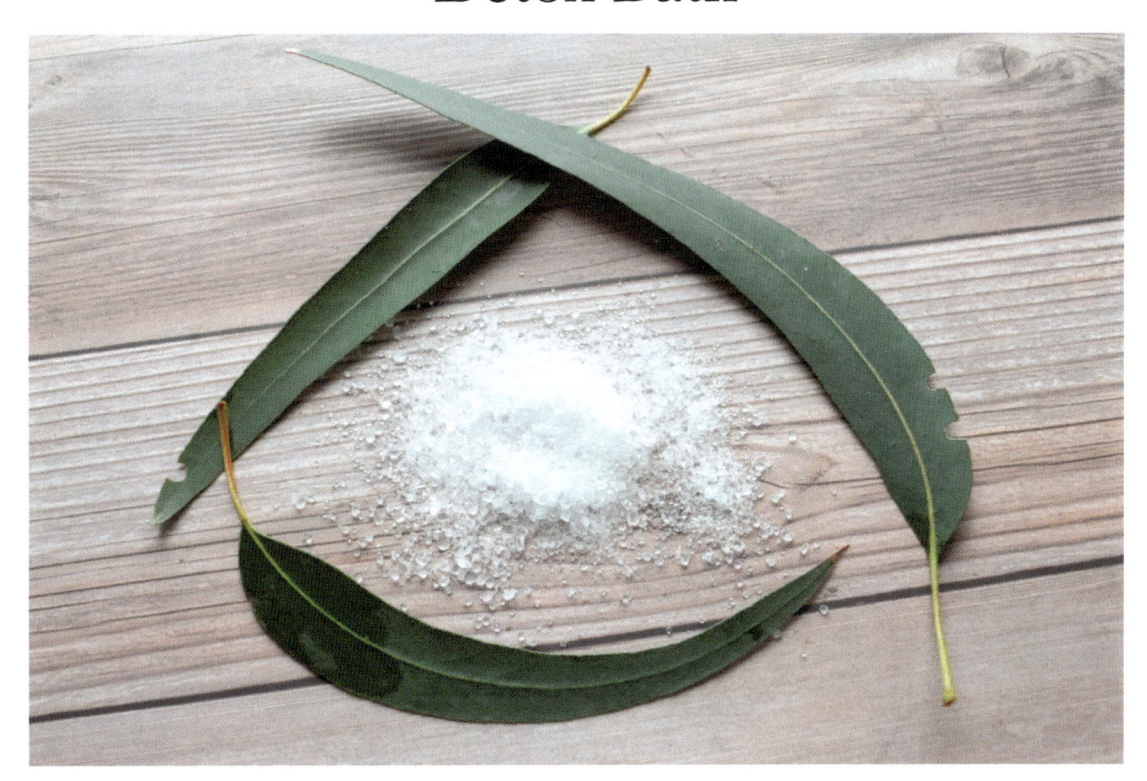

Ingredients:

2 cups of Epsom salts
1 cup of apple cider vinegar
1/2 cup of Bentonite clay
5-10 drops of eucalyptus essential oil.

Directions:

Add all the above ingredients to warm water in your bath tub. Soak for 20 minutes.

Benefits:

It is good to detox our bodies every now and then. This recipe will help, plus, you will get the benefits from the Epsom salts and vinegar. There is magnesium and sulfate in Epsom salts which is absorbed through the skin, it reduces inflammation and flushes toxins. The salts also work well to relax the body and remove stiffness in the muscles. Apple cider is good for the skin and may reduce blood pressure. It also has natural antibacterial properties. Eucalyptus is purifying and it has antibacterial, anti-fungal and antiseptic properties.

Natural Baby Powder

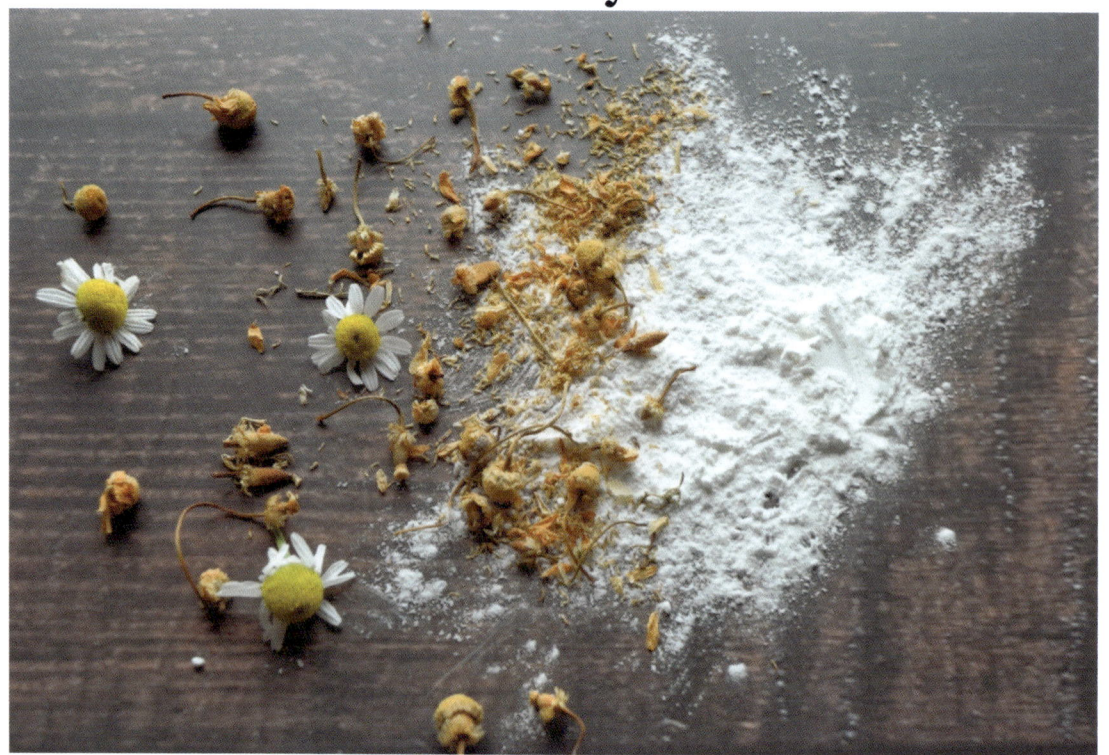

Ingredients:

1 oz white clay
1 tablespoon dried German chamomile flowers finely ground into a powder
1 tablespoon arrow root
1 teaspoon vanilla bean powder
20 drops of chamomile essential oil.

Directions:

Add all of the dry ingredients to a large bowl and whisk slowly. As you mix slowly add one or two drops of the essential oil at a time until all of the oil is incorporated. (you don't want the powder to create a cloud over the bowl and you don't want to breath in the powder, wear a face mask). Put it into a powder shaker.

How to use: This can be used for babies, children and adults. Gently shake the container to apply powder to the body anywhere it is needed.

Benefits:

Unlike the store bought powders this one does not have any chemicals. White clay absorbs oil and moisture. Arrow root keeps from chafing. The chamomile essential oil and flowers are mild, soothing and it has relaxing properties. It has wonderful skin healing properties, which include helping to tone skin, it is good for rashes, and it softens the skin and acts as an anti inflammatory. The essential oil is also good for sensitive skin. It is calming and soothing. The vanilla bean powder compliments the chamomile and makes the powder smell nice.

Natural Bug Spray

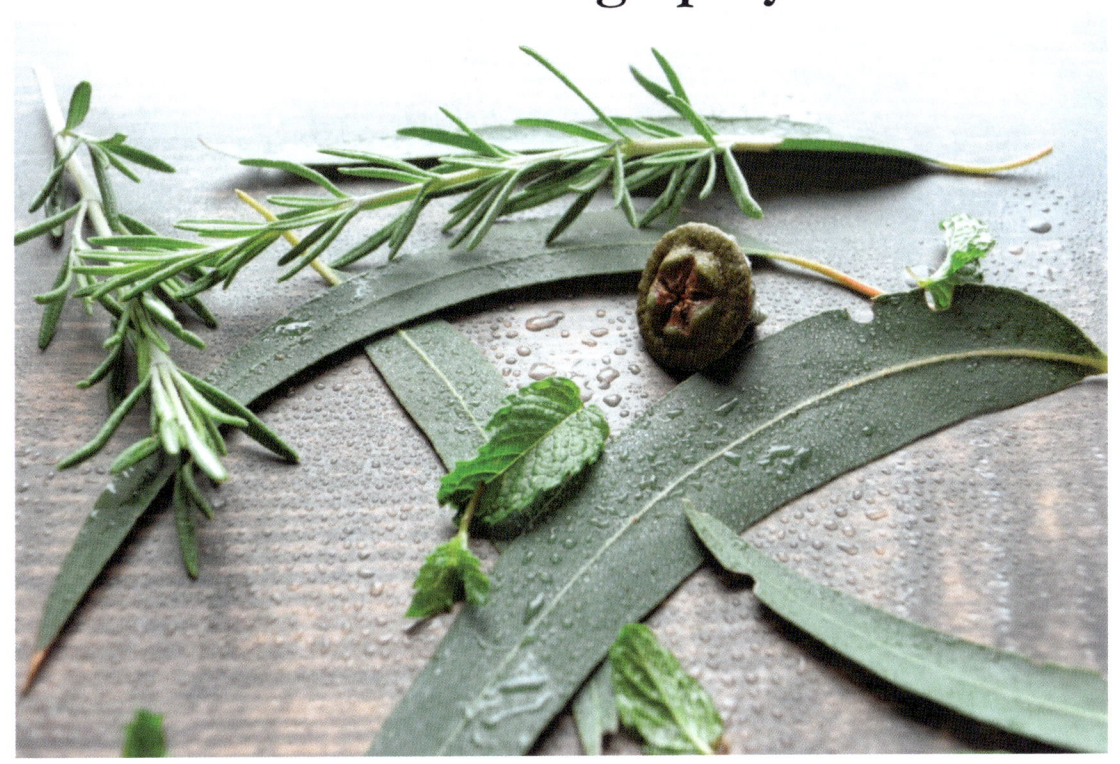

Ingredients:

4 drops citronella essential oil
4 drops rosemary essential oil
4 drops eucalyptus essential oil
4 drops of cedar wood essential oil
4 drops peppermint essential oil
1/4 cup witch hazel
small spray bottle

Directions:

Add all ingredients into a small spray bottle.

How to use:

Shake well and apply liberally to your clothes and bare skin. Reapply every two hours.

Benefits:

Citronella essential oil slows the spread of harmful airborne bacteria, and repels flying insects. Rosemary is an ancient herb that has been used for thousands for years. The strong scent can repel bugs. It is anti-fungal, and an insecticide. Cedar wood essential oil works well for a bug repellent because of the strong scent. Peppermint has a very strong odor and it is offensive to insects.

Soothing and Softening Foot Soak

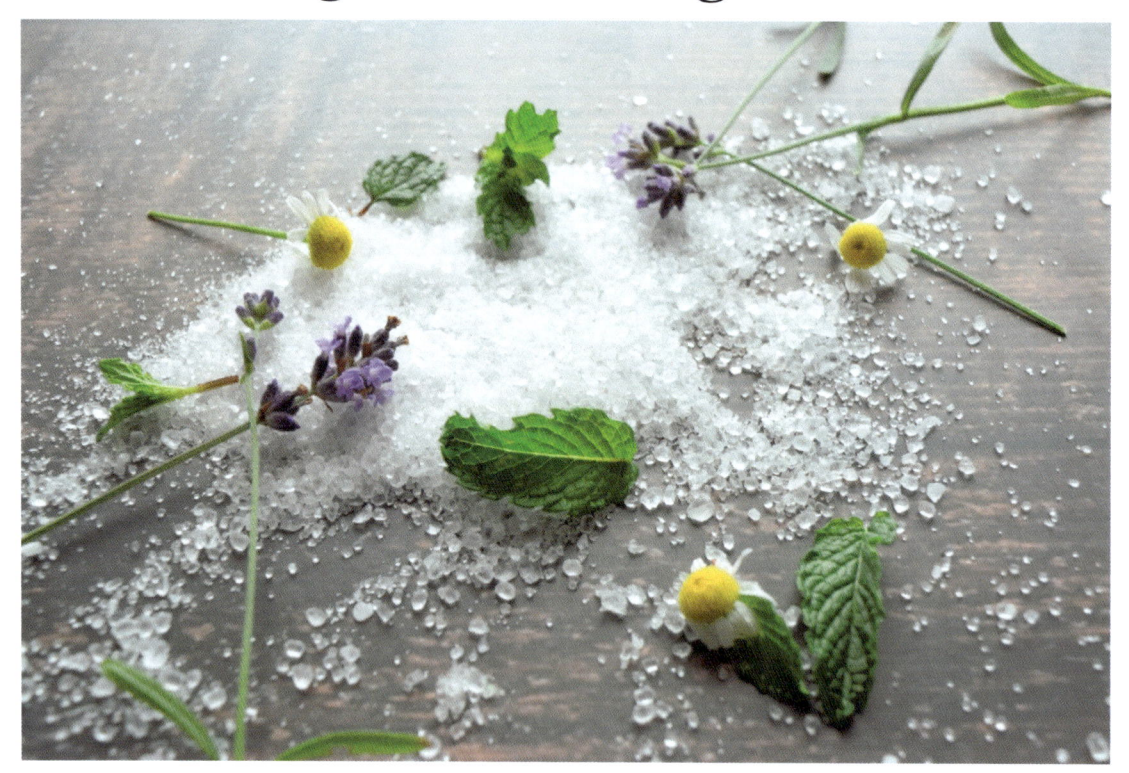

Ingredients:

2 tablespoons Epsom salt
2 tablespoons baking soda
3 drops peppermint essential oil
3 drops lavender essential oil
3 drops chamomile essential oil
1 gallon of very warm water

Directions: Mix all of the ingredients in a bowl then dissolve into a basin of warm water and soak feet until water is cool.

Benefits:

Epsom salts which is absorbed through the skin reduces inflammation and flushes toxins. The salts also work well to relax the body and remove stiffness in the muscles. Baking soda is not only a good exfoliator but also helps by slightly shrinking the size of your pores, thereby preventing dirt and other particulate matter from clogging them. There are anti-bacterial and anti-inflammatory properties of baking soda. It can make your skin soft too. Peppermint essential oil has anti-inflammatory and astringent properties. It's vitalizing and refreshing it energizes the mind and body. Mint also helps clean pores. It has a powerful sweet crisp scent. It relieves muscle and joint pain. It also has cooling, invigorating and has antispasmodic properties. Lavender essential oil has wonderful healing properties for the skin; it helps relieve itchy skin and acne. Lavender essential oil has natural antibacterial and antidepressant properties. The fragrance revives your spirits. Chamomile has wonderful skin healing properties, which include helping to tone skin, it is good for rashes, and it softens the skin and acts as an anti inflammatory. The essential oil is also good for sensitive skin. It is calming and soothing.

Peppermint and Tea Tree Foot Soak

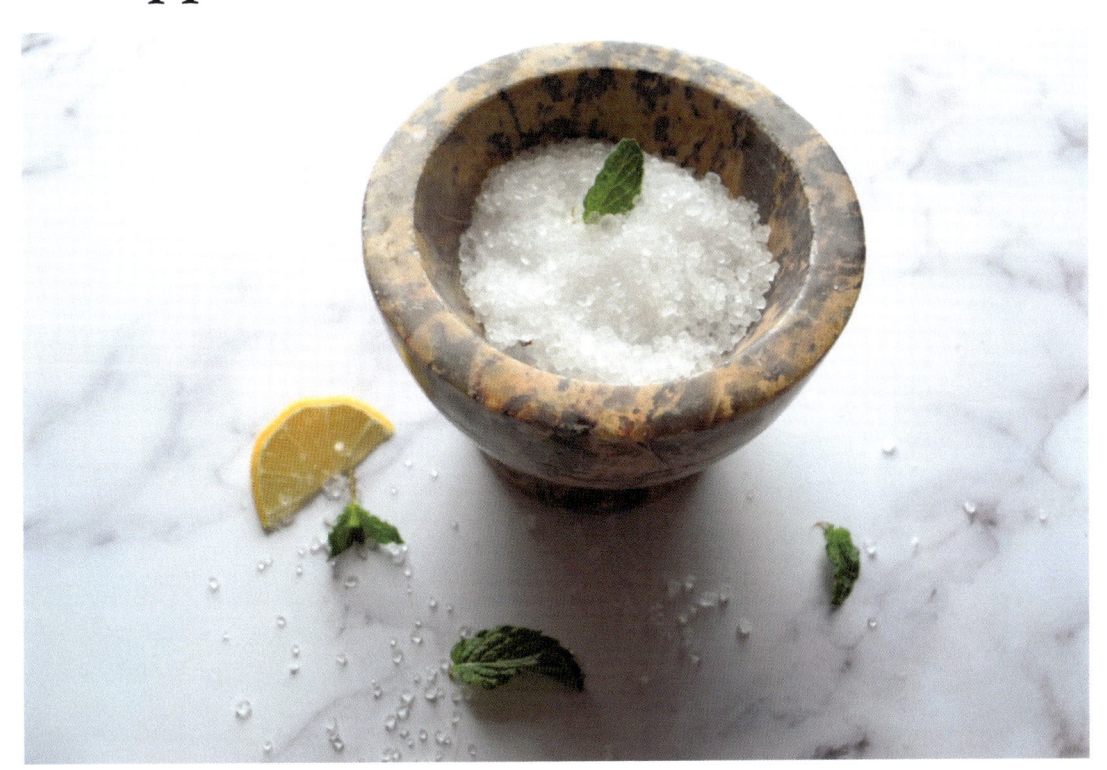

Ingredients:

1/2 gallon warm water
1/2 cup Epsom salt
1 tablespoon baking soda
juice of 1/2 fresh lemon, or about 1 tbsp. lemon juice
2 tablespoons of olive oil
20 drops peppermint essential oil
10 drops of tea tree essential oil
plastic tub for foot soak

Directions: In a small cup mix the olive oil and essential oil together. Warm 1/2 gallon of water to a comfortable temperature and pour it into a foot bath tub. Add the lemon juice, Epsom salt, and baking soda to the warm water, and stir to dissolve. Next add the olive oil and essential oil, and stir to mix well.

How to use: Soak your feet for 15 minutes. Do not store any leftovers it will not keep well.

Benefits:

Epsom salts which is absorbed through the skin reduces inflammation and flushes toxins. The salts also work well to relax the body and remove stiffness in the muscles. Baking soda is not only a good exfoliator but also helps by slightly shrinking the size of your pores, thereby preventing dirt and other particulate matter from clogging them. There are anti-bacterial and anti-inflammatory properties of baking soda. It can make your skin soft too. Peppermint essential oil has anti-inflammatory and astringent properties. It's vitalizing and refreshing it energizes the mind and body. Mint also helps clean pores. It has a powerful sweet crisp scent. It relieves muscle and joint pain. It also has cooling, invigorating and antispasmodic properties. Tea Tree essential oil has natural antibacterial and anti-inflammatory properties.

Hand Sanitizer

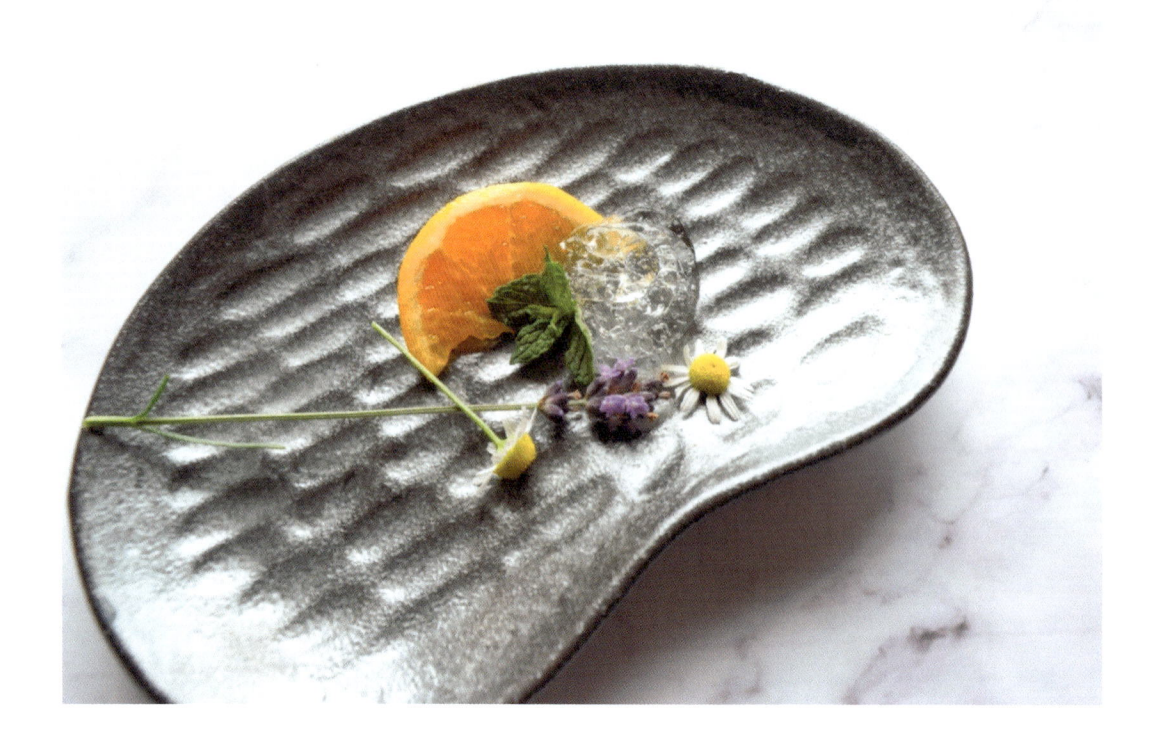

Ingredients:

4 oz organic aloe vera gel
4 drops peppermint essential oil
8 drops lavender essential oil
8 drops orange essential oil
1 ounce of rubbing alcohol
4 oz plastic squeeze bottle

Directions:

Add oils to the aloe vera gel and alcohol in a bottle and shake vigorously to combine.

How to use:

Apply liberally to hands and rub until the gel has evaporated. This can be stored in the fridge and transferred into convenient 1 oz squeeze bottles to keep in your purse or diaper bag for hand sanitizing on the go. Avoid purchasing aloe with extra ingredients a small amount of natural preservative is fine.

Benefits:

Lavender oil is believed to have antiseptic and anti-inflammatory properties. Peppermint oil and menthol have moderate antibacterial effects peppermint is also found to possess antiviral and fungicidal activities. Orange essential has natural antimicrobial properties. Rubbing alcohol kills germs and disinfects. Aloe vera gel softens skin and works as carrier of all of the ingredients.

Re-hydration Drink

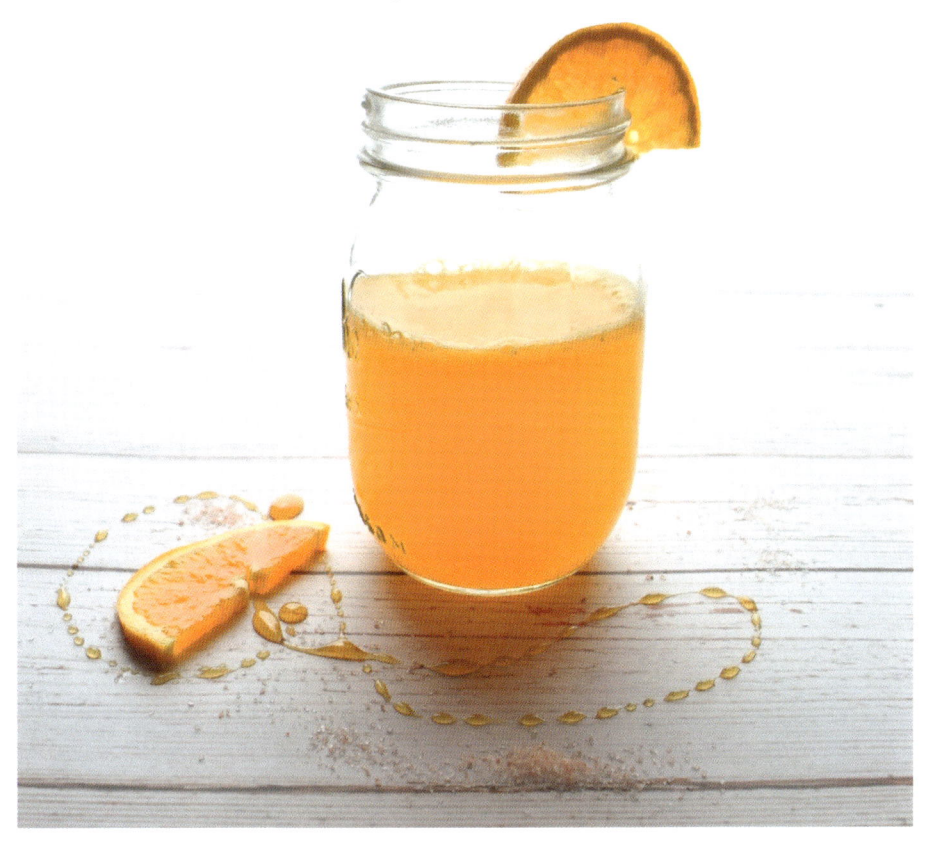

Ingredients:

1/2 cup honey
1/2 teaspoon sea salt
2 cups orange juice
5 1/2 cups water

Directions:

Place all ingredients in a bottle or mason jar with a lid, shake well to mix honey.

How to use:

Drink throughout the day to energize and rehydrate your body.

Benefits:

Drinks containing some carbohydrate in the form of sugars and electrolytes, usually sodium, can be absorbed by the body more quickly than pure water and therefore allow re-hydration to happen more rapidly. The honey acts as the carbohydrate and the salt acts as the electrolyte. The orange provides vitamin C and potassium which is important if you are dehydrated.

Cold Care Drink

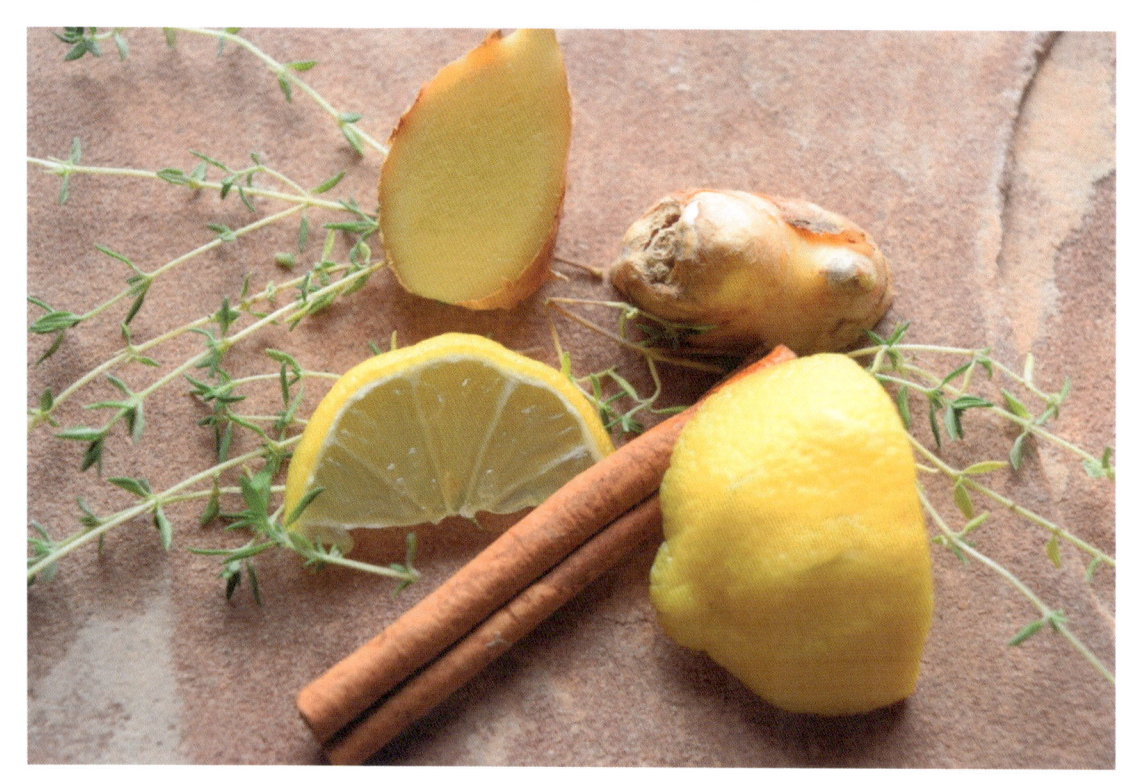

Ingredients:

1 lemon cut into slices
1/2 cinnamon stick
3 sprigs fresh thyme roughly chopped
3 tablespoons fresh grated ginger
3 teaspoons honey
3-4 cups boiling water

Directions:

Put all of the ingredients into a small sauce pan and simmer for 10 minutes.

To use:

Drink 4-5 ounces at a time throughout the day. You can drink it warm or cold.

Benefits:

Lemon is full of vitamin C which will boost your immunity and help you feel better. Cinnamon contains potent antibacterial, antiviral, analgesic and anti-inflammatory properties. Thyme has antiviral, antibiotic, antimicrobial, decongestant, and expectorant properties that help fight off or reduce the time you are sick with a cold or flu. Thyme can strengthen the immune system. Ginger is also believed to have antimicrobial properties that may help fight infections (bacterial or viral), including those that cause sore throat. Honey has antimicrobial properties, which may allow it to fight some bacteria and viruses.

Eucalyptus Steam for the Sinuses

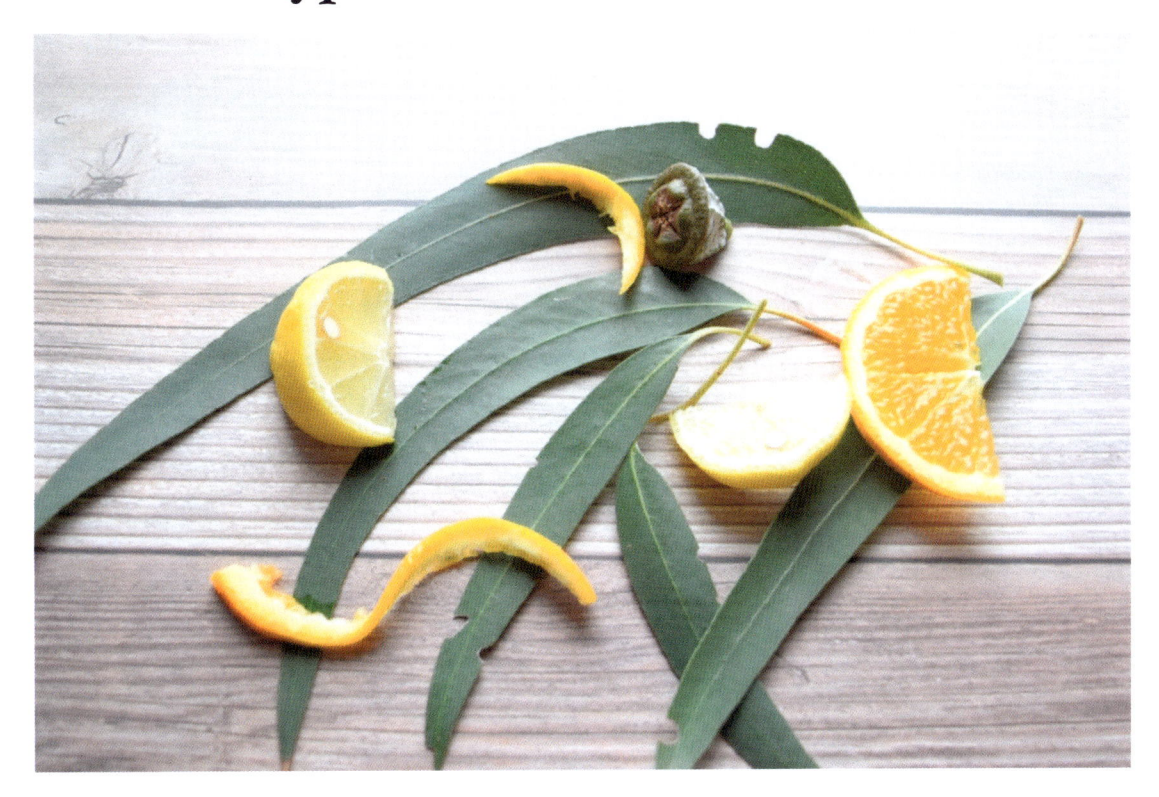

Ingredients:

4 drops eucalyptus essential oil
2 drops lemon essential oil
1 drop tea tree essential oil
1 drop orange essential oil
4-6 cups of boiling water
a large towel

Directions and use:

Bring water to boil and pour into a 1 to 3 quart mixing bowl. Drop in your essential oils. With your head positioned over the bowl, drape the towel over your head and shoulders to create a steam-catching tent. Close your eyes and breathe in the vapor. Do not put your face too close to the stream. If the vapor gets too hot, just lift a corner of the towel when you need to get a little cool air. Continue breathing deeply for as long as you like, or until the water is no longer releasing steam.

Benefits:

This blend is helpful for moistening the breathing passages and is wonderfully soothing. Eucalyptus essential oil has antibacterial, anti-fungal and antiseptic properties. The scent helps to open the sinuses. The lemon, lavender and orange essential oils all have antimicrobial, antibacterial and antiviral properties to help heal your sinuses. Tea tree is a powerful antibacterial and has a strong scent that will help open your sinuses.

Elderberry Syrup

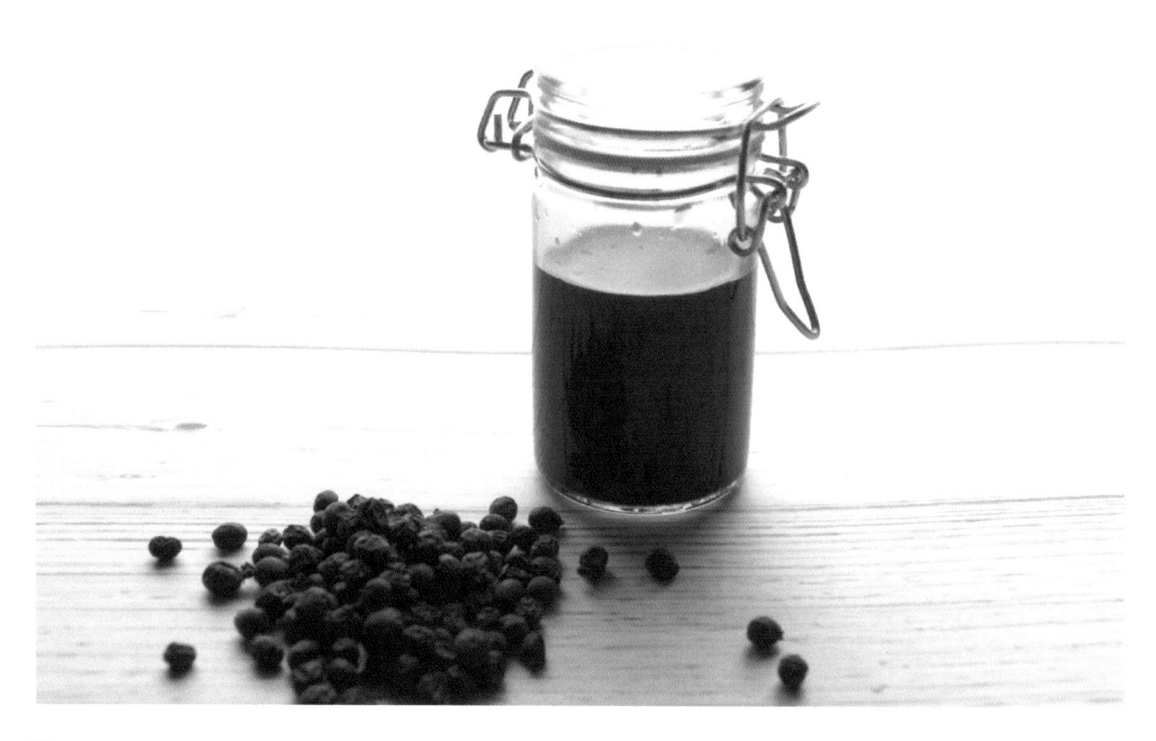

Ingredients

2/3 cup dried elderberries
3 cups water
1 teaspoon ground cinnamon
1/2 teaspoon ground clove
1/2 teaspoon ground ginger
1 cup honey raw
2/3 cup raw apple cider vinegar

Directions: Simmer berries, spices and water in a sauce pot, stirring occasionally until liquid is reduced by half about 45 minutes. Strain liquid into a bowl using a colander or strainer and discard elderberries. Mix in honey and then add apple cider vinegar mixing well. Let cool then pour into clean glass jar and refrigerate for up to 3 months.

How to use: Standard dose for cold and flu prevention: 1 tsp daily for kids and 1 tbsp daily for adults. If you are sick, take the above dose every 2-3 hours as needed.

Benefits: Elderberries and flowers of elderberry tree are packed with antioxidants and vitamins that may boost your immune system. They can help tame inflammation, lessen stress, and help protect your heart too. Some experts recommend elderberry to help prevent and ease cold and flu symptoms. Honey contains an array of plant chemicals that act as antioxidants. Some types of honey have as many antioxidants as fruits and vegetables. Antioxidants help to protect your body from cell damage due to free radicals. The phytonutrients in honey are responsible for its antioxidant properties, as well as its antibacterial and anti-fungal power. They're also thought to be the reason raw honey has shown immune-boosting benefits. Cinnamon is high in antioxidants. Cinnamon is packed with a variety of protective antioxidants that reduce free radical damage and slow the aging process. Ginger may have anti-inflammatory, antibacterial, antiviral, and other healthful properties.

Golden Milk

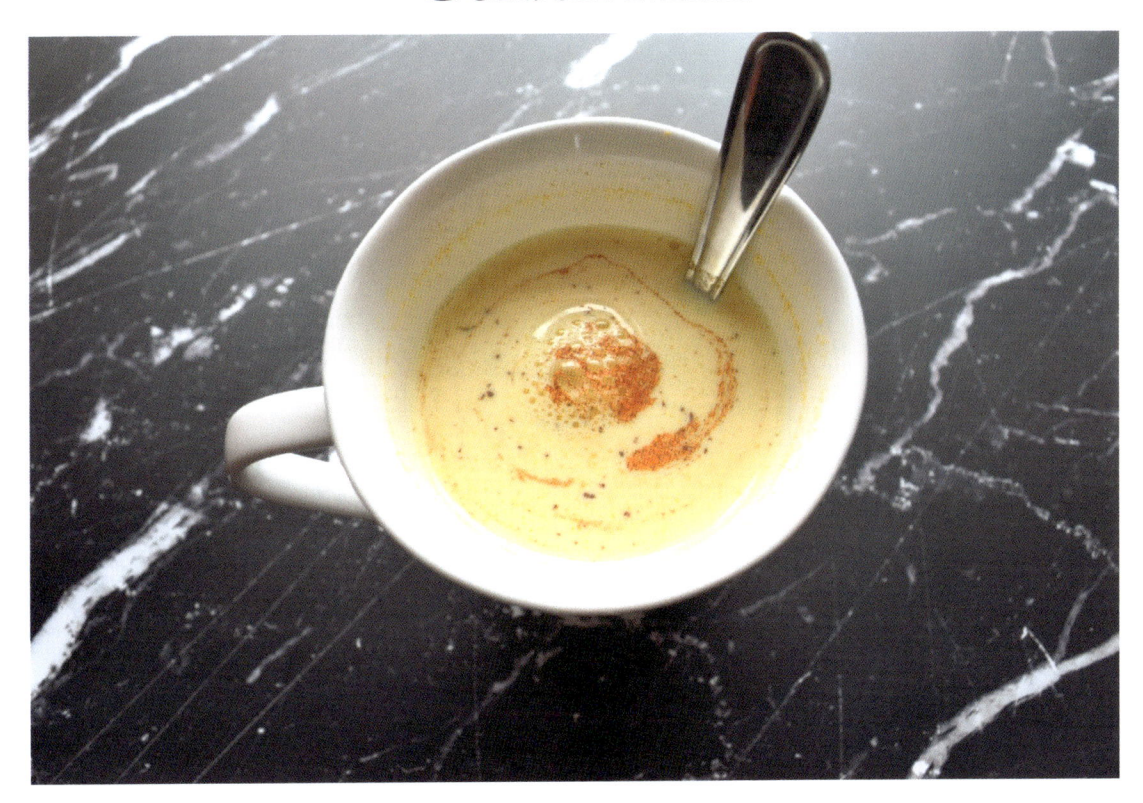

Ingredients:

2 cups of regular milk, soy milk, almond or rice milk
1 teaspoon of ground turmeric
1 tablespoon of honey
1 teaspoon of ground ginger
1/2 teaspoon of cinnamon

Directions: In a small saucepan add the milk and bring to almost a boil then add the honey and spices mix well. Simmer on low for 2 minutes. Makes 2 cups.

How to use: Drink one cup before bed.

Benefits:

The compounds in turmeric are called curcuminoids, the most important of which is curcumin. Curcumin is the main active ingredient in turmeric. It has powerful anti-inflammatory effects and is a very strong antioxidant. Cinnamon is high in antioxidants. Cinnamon is packed with a variety of protective antioxidants that reduce free radical damage and slow the aging process. Ginger may have anti-inflammatory, antibacterial, antiviral, and other healthful properties. Honey contains an array of plant chemicals that act as antioxidants. Antioxidants help to protect your body from cell damage due to free radicals. The phytonutrients in honey are responsible for its antioxidant properties, as well as its antibacterial and anti-fungal power. Honey may have immune-boosting benefits.

Healthy Tea Mixes

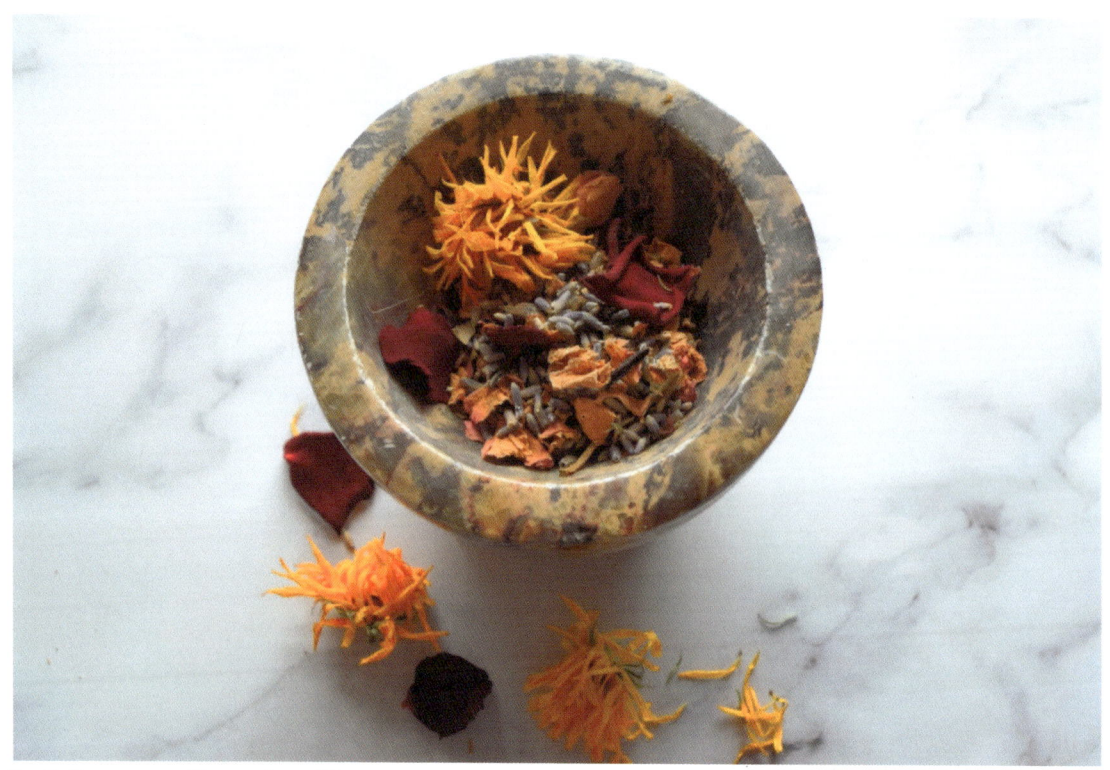

High-C Immune Boosting Tea
This tea is great year around. Hibiscus with its lovely tart flavor and pretty red coloring and is rich in vitamin C, helping to boost your immunities.
1 part hibiscus
1 part rose hips
1/2 part lemon grass
1/2 part lemon peel
1/4 part cinnamon chips

Headache Relief Tea
This tea is great for relieving headaches, easing tension, calming nausea, and even for helping aid in sleep.
1 part basil leaf
1 part lemon balm
1/4 part chamomile
1/4 part lavender

No Nausea Tea
This tea is great for nausea, upset stomach, and indigestion.
1 part lemon balm
1 part chamomile
1 part peppermint leaf
1 part ginger powder

Directions: Combine the dried herbs in a bowl and store in a sealed container when not in use.
To make a medicinal infusion add 4-6 tablespoons in a tea pot or a large mug and pour hot water over the tea and let steep for 5 minutes. Strain the herbs and drink the tea.

Fire Cider

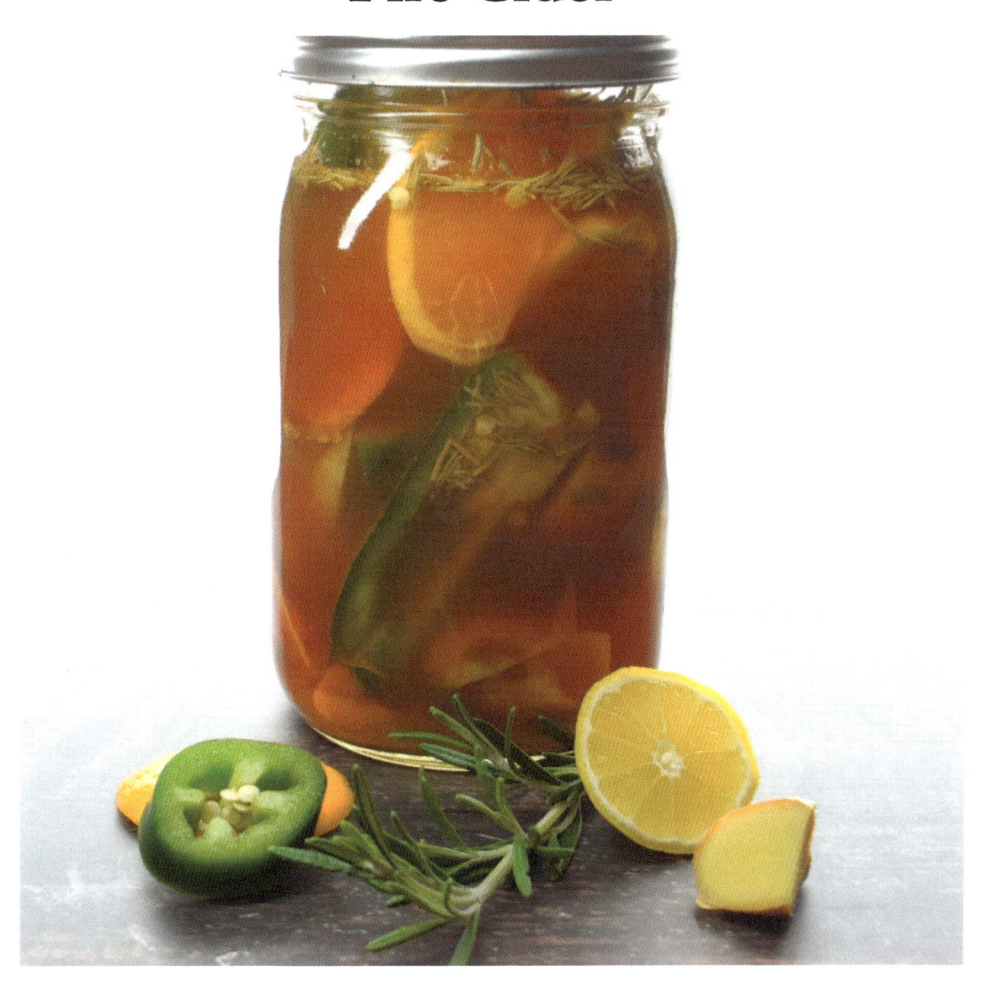

Ingredients:

1 medium onion, chopped
10 cloves of garlic, crushed or chopped
2 jalapeño peppers, chopped
1 whole lemon sliced
1/2 cup fresh grated ginger root
1/2 cup fresh grated horseradish root
1 tablespoon turmeric powder
1/4 teaspoon cayenne powder
1 tablespoon of cinnamon
2 tablespoon of dried rosemary leaves
1-2 cups apple cider vinegar
1/4 cup of honey
1 small orange cut up
1 quart Mason jar with a plastic lid

Directions: Prepare your roots, fruits, and herbs and place them in the quart-sized glass jar. If you've never grated fresh horseradish, be prepared for a powerful sinus-opening experience! Pour the apple cider vinegar in the jar until all of the ingredients are covered and the vinegar reaches the jar's top put the cover on. Shake well. Store in a dark, cool place for a month and remember to shake daily. After a month, use cheesecloth to strain out the pulp, pour the cider into a clean jar. Be sure to squeeze as much of the liquid out as you can. Then add the honey and stir until well blended.

How to use: Take 1 tablespoon daily.

Benefits: Fire Cider is said to strengthen the immune system, it is full of nutrients and vitamins that nourish the body. It can aid your digestion, and ease sinus congestion.
There is a reason it's called "FIRE" Cider, it has some potent and spicy ingredients!

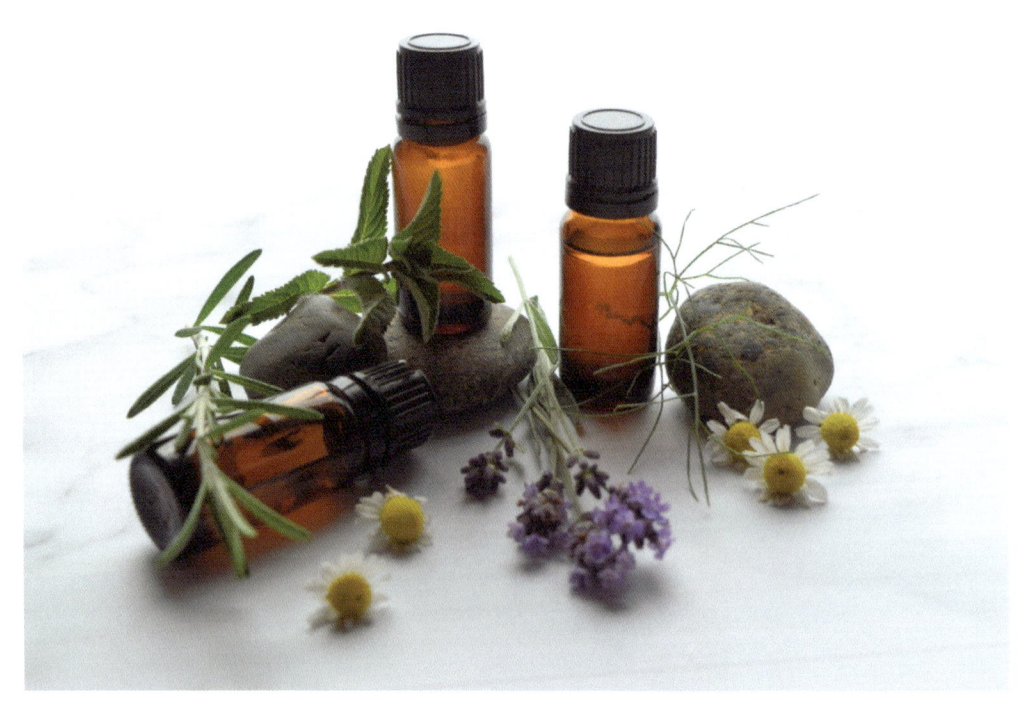

Easy Aromatherapy

In this section you will find simple and easy Aromatherapy. Got a headache and don't want to take any medication? Rosemary is the go to essential oil for headaches. You will learn how essential oils can benefit your body and give you some relief from everyday issues. Buying quality essential oils is important. Be careful that you only get therapeutic grade essential oils. I have included some good sources at the end of the book of where you can find essential oils. Also do not ingest any essential oils without a health care provider's supervision or advice.

Commuter's Aromatherapy Spray

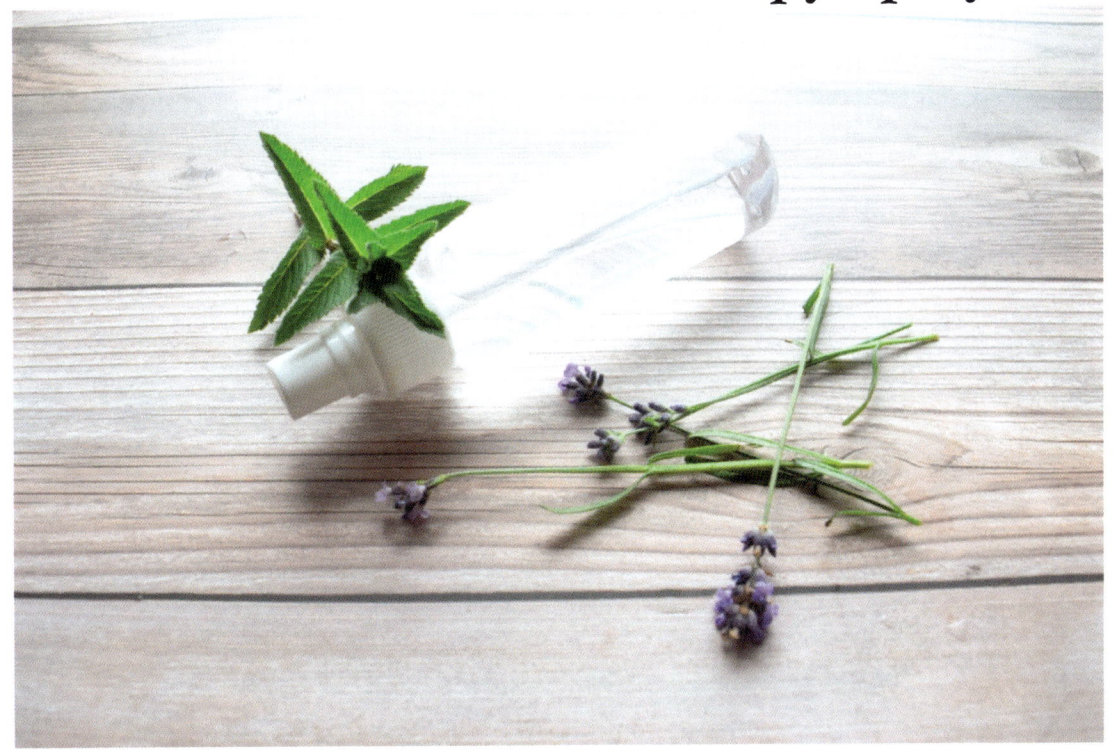

Ingredients:

2 oz. distilled water
6 drops lavender essential oil
2 drops Clary sage essential oil
2 drops geranium essential oil
2 drops peppermint essential oil
small spray bottle

Directions and use:

Combine oils and water in spray bottle and shake well. Spray throughout the vehicle before you drive.

Benefits:

Lavender essential oil aromatherapy benefits: balancing, soothing, normalizing, calming, relaxing, and healing. Clary Sage essential oil aromatherapy benefits: centering, euphoric, visualizing. Geranium essential oil aromatherapy benefits: soothing, mood-lifting, balancing. Peppermint essential oil aromatherapy benefits: vitalizing, refreshing, and cooling.

Positivity Aromatherapy Mist

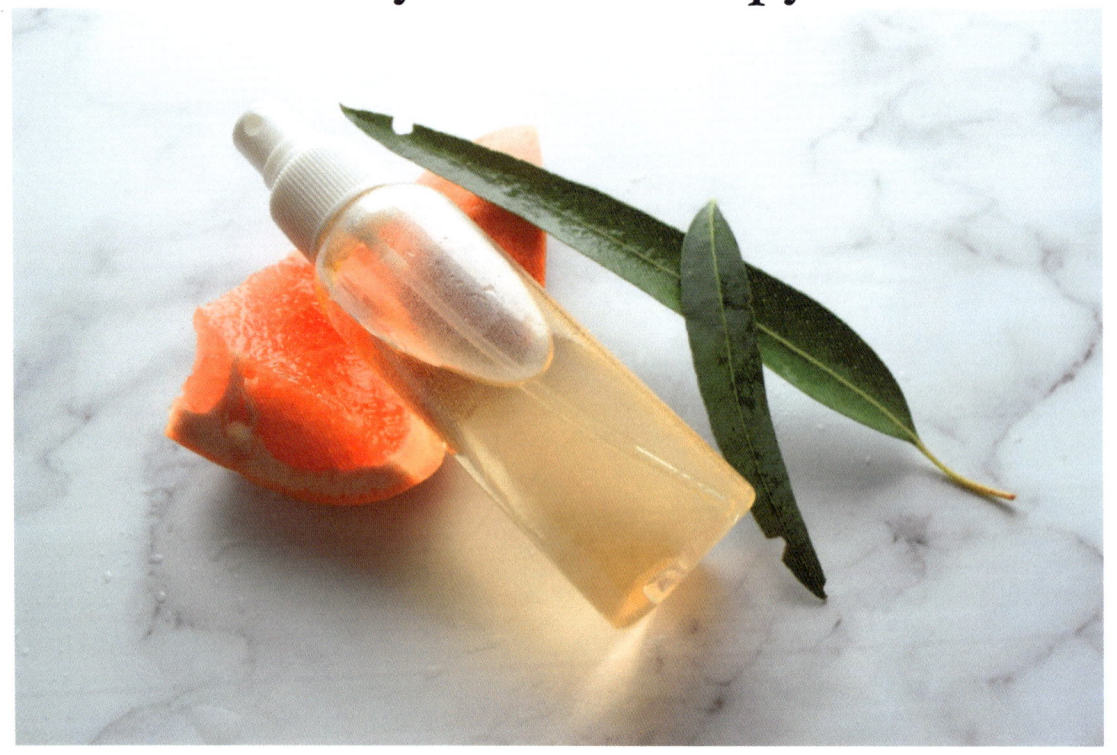

Ingredients:

4 ounces water
12 drops bergamot essential oil
6 drops grapefruit essential oil
6 drops eucalyptus essential oil
small spray bottle

Directions:

Place ingredients in a spray bottle, shake well.

How to use:

Mist the air to create an aura of positivity.

Benefits:

Bergamot is uplifting, inspiring and confidence building. Grapefruit is refreshing and cheering. The essential oil of grapefruit is said to be an anti-depressant because it has a cheering and refreshing fragrance. Eucalyptus is purifying, invigorating.

Headache Aromatherapy Roll On

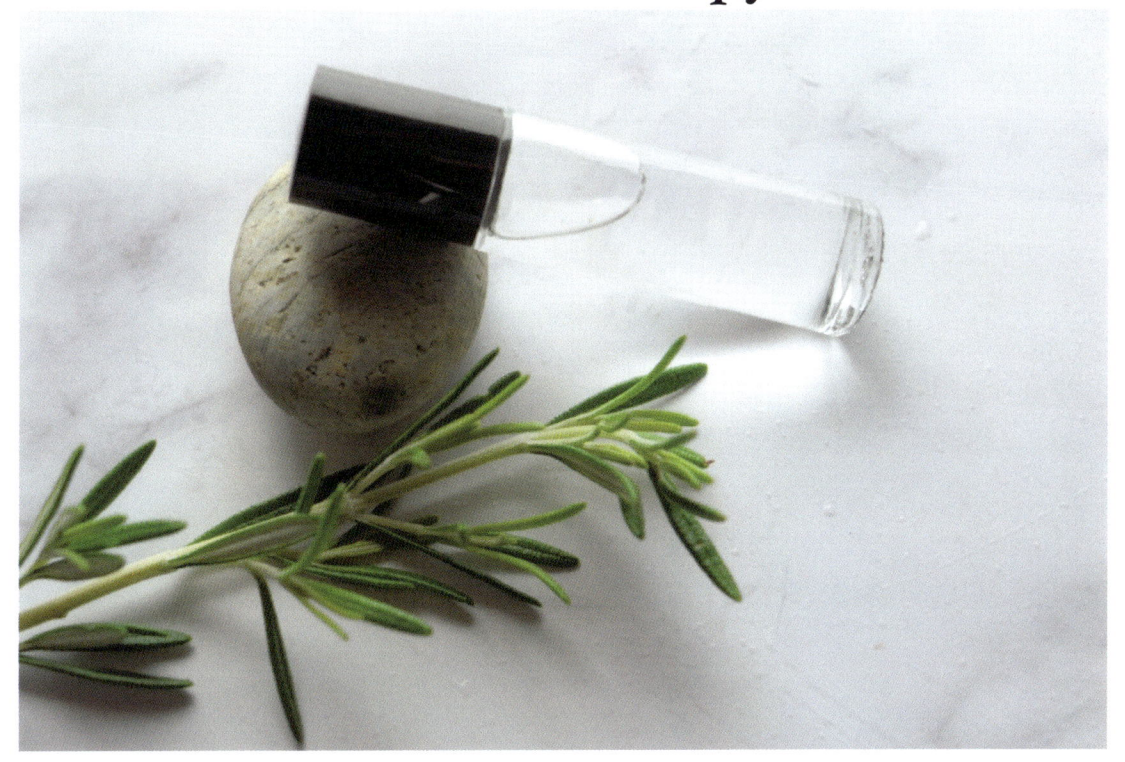

Ingredients:

.5 ounce of olive oil or rice bran oil
20 drops of rosemary essential oil
glass roll on bottle

Directions:

Add the olive oil to the roll on bottle and then add the rosemary essential oil. Put roller top on then the cap and shake well.

How to use:

When you have a headache or need a clear head for studying roll onto your forehead two times and the back of the neck two times.

Benefits:

Rosemary essential oil has pain relieving properties, it also stimulates blood flow which can relive headaches and help with memory.

Aromatherapy Inhalers

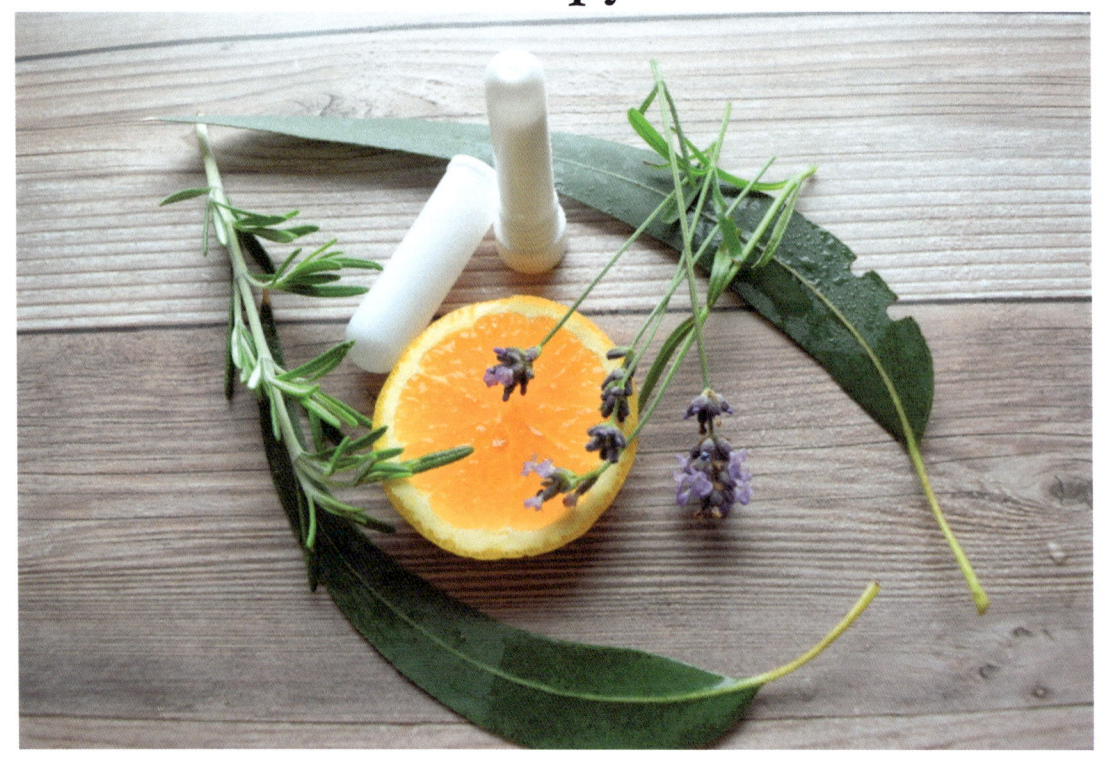

Calm

Add 20 drops of lavender essential oil to the cotton in the nasal inhaler tube.

Aromatherapy benefits: balancing, soothing, normalizing, calming, relaxing, and healing.

Headache

Add 20 drops of rosemary essential oil to the cotton in the nasal inhaler tube.

Aromatherapy benefits: Rosemary stimulates circulation and relieves headaches.

Stuffy nose

Add 20 drops of eucalyptus essential oil to the cotton in the nasal inhaler tube.

Aromatherapy benefits: It works to open the sinuses. It is purifying, invigorating.

Cheer up

Add 20 drops of orange essential oil to the cotton in the nasal inhaler tube.

Aromatherapy benefits: cheering, refreshing, uplifting.

To use: open inhaler and hold tip to your nose and inhale deeply, repeat on the other side. Use as often as needed.

Sleep Aromatherapy Roll On

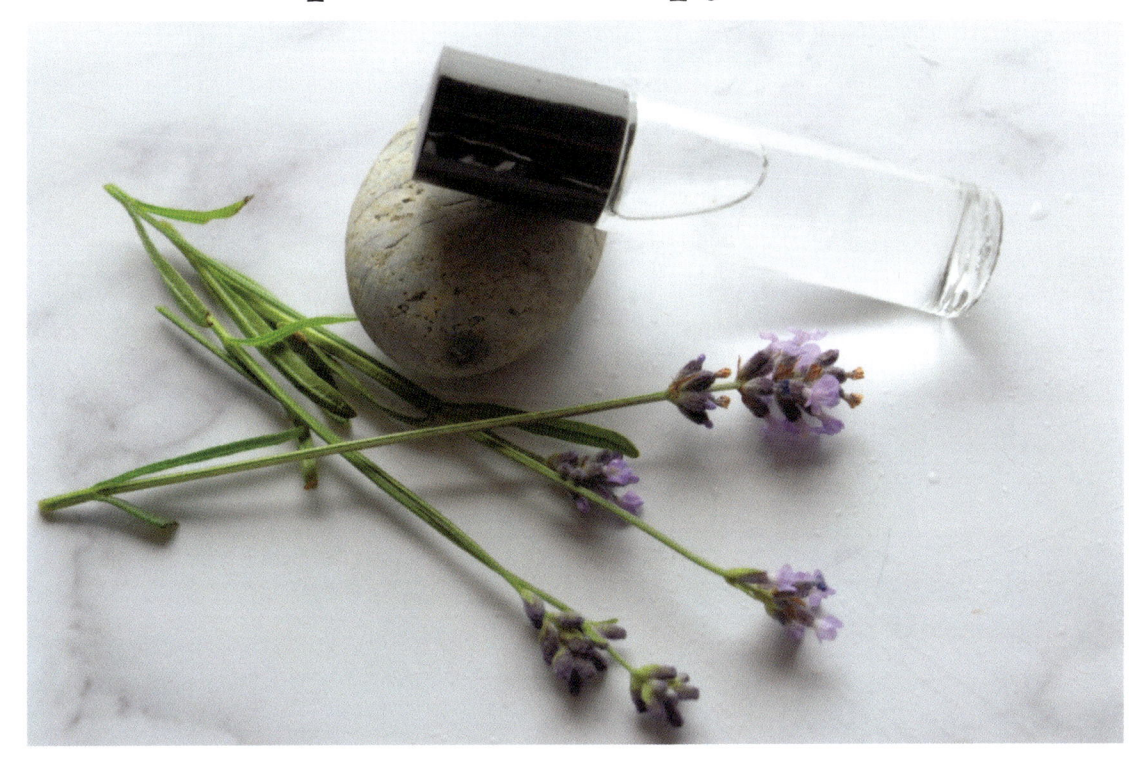

Ingredients:

.5 ounce of olive oil or rice bran oil
20 drops of lavender essential oil
glass roll on bottle

Directions:

Add the olive oil to the roll on bottle and then add the lavender essential oil. Put roller top on then the cap and shake well.

How to use:

When you can't sleep roll onto your forehead two times and the back of the neck two times.

Benefits:

Balancing, soothing, normalizing, calming, relaxing, and healing. Lavender can help you sleep.

Be Happy Aromatherapy Spray

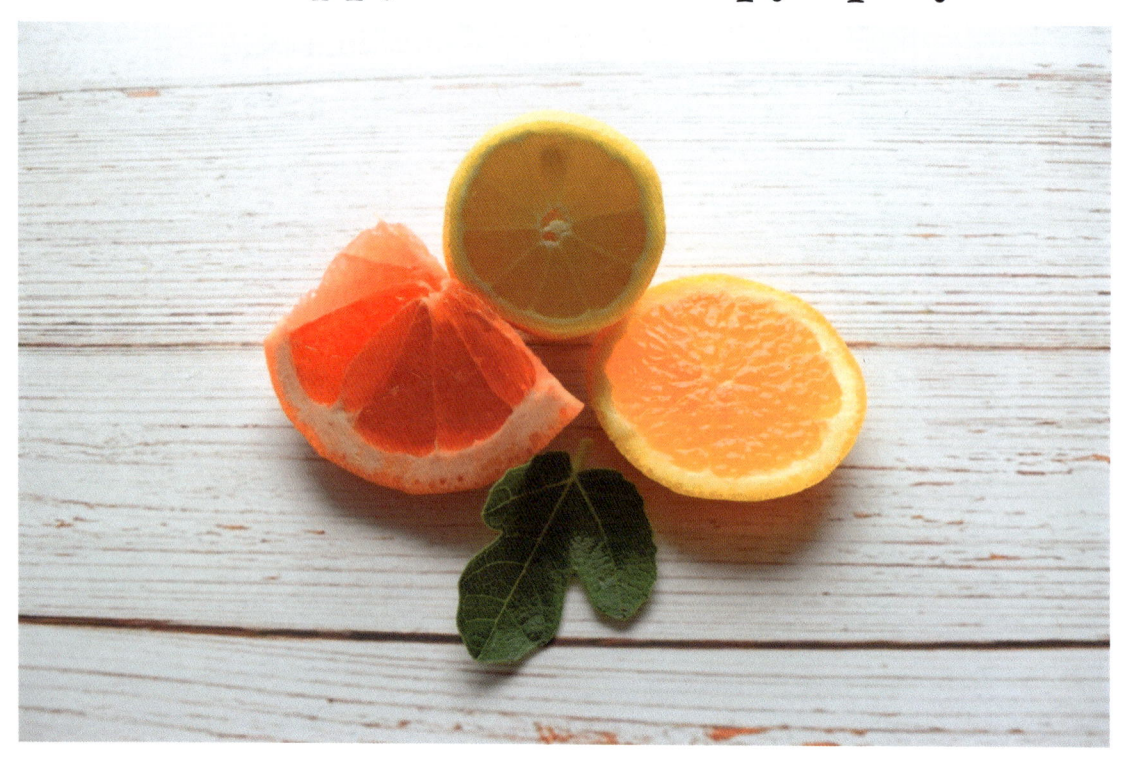

Ingredients:

4 ounces of water
12 drops of orange essential oil
12 drops of grapefruit essential oil
12 drops of lemon essential oil
small spray bottle

Directions:

Place water and essential oils in spray bottle. Shake contents and mist the air throughout your area to help you feel happy.

Benefits:

Lemon essential oil aromatherapy benefits: uplifting, refreshing, and cheering.
Orange essential oil aromatherapy benefits: cheering, refreshing, uplifting.
Grapefruit essential oil aromatherapy benefits: refreshing, cheering.

Purifying Aromatherapy Air Freshener

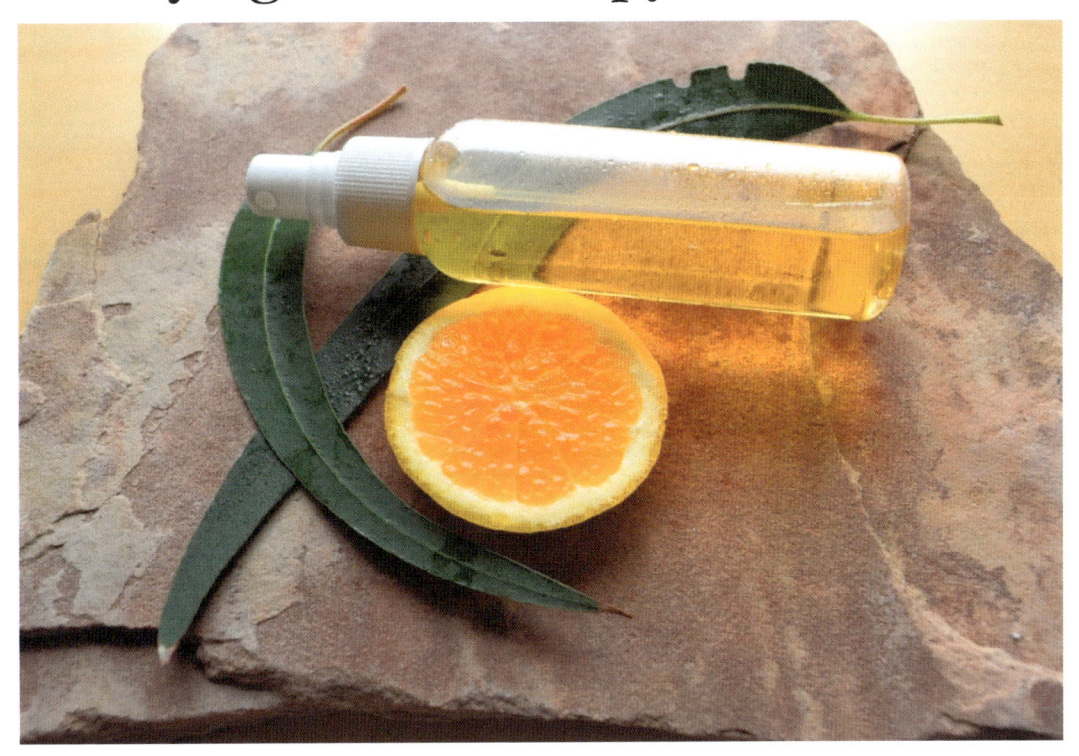

Ingredients:

4 ounces water
12 drops sweet orange essential oil
6 drops eucalyptus essential oil
6 drops pine essential oil
4 ounce spray bottle

Directions:

Place water and essential oils in spray bottle. Shake contents and mist the air throughout your home to purify the air.

Benefits:

Orange essential oil aromatherapy benefits: cheering, refreshing, uplifting.

Eucalyptus essential oil aromatherapy benefits: purifying, invigorating. Pine essential oil aromatherapy benefits: refreshing, invigorating

Herbal Sleep Pillow

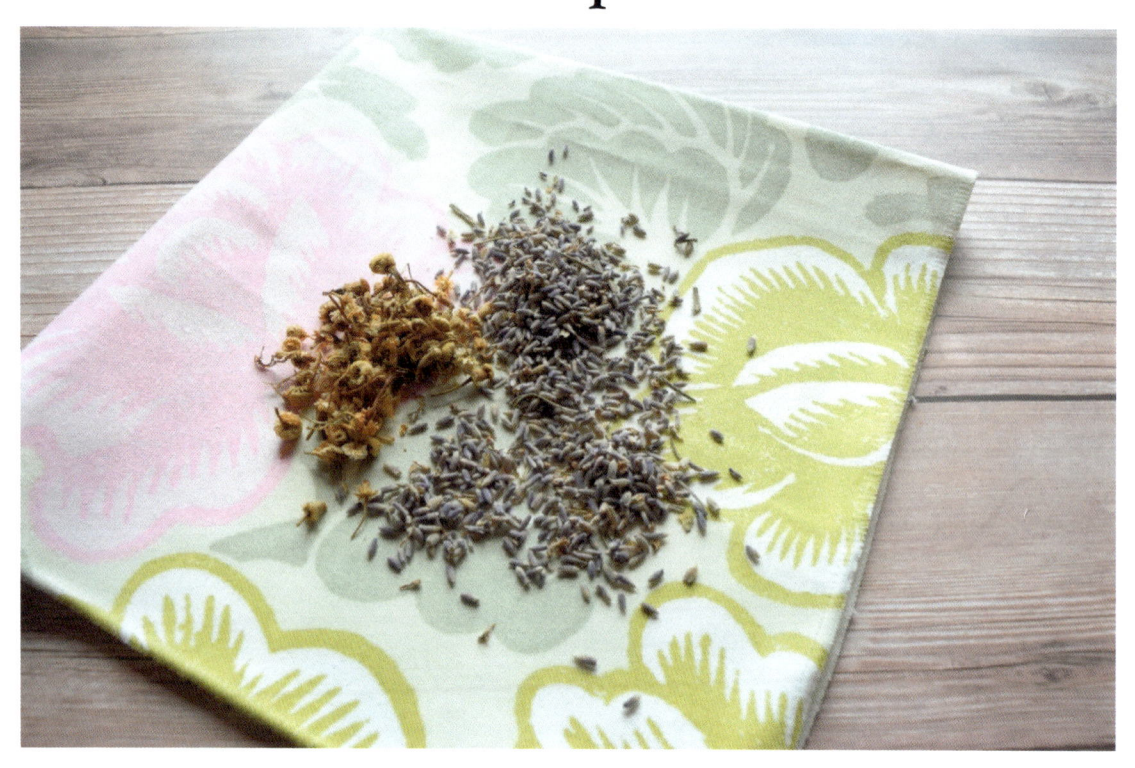

Ingredients:

2 cups of dried lavender buds
1 cup dried chamomile flowers
2 squares of 8x8 inch fabric preferably cotton
20 drops of essential oil lavender essential oil
20 drops of chamomile essential oil
thread and needle or a sewing machine.

Directions:

Sew the fabric together using small stitches. Leave a 2 inch hole at one of the corners. In a bowl mix the lavender buds and chamomile buds with the essential oils. Fill the pillow through the hole you left near the corner. When you are done filling the pillow sew up the hole. If you have some dried buds left, you can put them in a small jar or bowl and leave it next to your bed.

To use:

Crush the pillow right before you go to sleep and lay the pillow next to you while you sleep. Crushing the pillow releases the essential oils so you can smell them.

Benefits: Lavender and Chamomile promote sleep, calmness and relaxation.

Supplies resources
Mountainroseherbs.com - herbs
Amazon – 30% vinegar, Borax, Baking Soda, Castile Soap, Epsom Salts
Brambleberry.com – soap supplies, essential oils
Bulkapothecary.com –soap supplies, essential oils, herbs
fromnaturewithlove.com- essential oils, herbs
Wholefoods Grocery Store, Castile Soap
Sprouts Grocery Store, Castile Soap
SKS bottles- bottles and packaging
Information Sources

www.webmd.com
www.healthline.com
draxe.com
www.aromahead.com
Mountainroseherbs.com
medicalnewstoday.com
cupertinosoap.com
motherearthliving.com
auracacia.com
herbanlifestyle.wordpress.com
Cultivating Medicinal Herbs.com
Book -Herbal Remedies, Andrew Chevallier
Book - The Complete Herbal Tutor, Anne McIntyre
Book - Your Backyard Herb Garden, Miranda Smith

Index

After shave pg 33
Air freshener pg 45
All purpose cleaner pg 47
Anti- aging face cream pg 19
Aromatherapy inhalers pg 82
Baby powder pg 66
Bath tub tea pg 31
Be happy aromatherapy spray pg 84
Bleach fee surface cleaning and disinfecting pg 42
Bug spray pg 67
Calendula ointment pg 62
Calendula rose hip facial serum pg 8
Calendula salve pg 63
Carpet cleaner machine solution #1 pg 56
Carpet cleaner machine solution #2 pg 57
Carpet freshener pg 55
Clay face mask pg 14
Coconut oil lotion bars pg 30
Coffee body scrub pg 20
Cold care drink pg 72
Commuter's aromatherapy spray pg 79
Cooling cucumber facial mask pg 16
Cuticle oil pg 35
Cuticle softener pg 36
Deep cleansing facial mud mask pg 13
Detox bath pg 65
Disinfectant wipes pg 52
Dry shampoo #1 pg 27
Dry shampoo #2 pg 28
Elderberry syrup pg 79
Eucalyptus steam for sinuses pg 73
Facial clay mask pg 15
Finger nail soak pg 37
Fire cider pg 77
Foot scrub pg 19
Foot soak pg 68
Golden milk pg 75
Green tea toner pg 10
Hand sanitizer pg 70
Headache aromatherapy roll on pg 81
Herbal sleep pillow pg 86
Holiday air freshener pg 44
Honey and olive oil hair conditioner pg 23
Laundry detergent #1 pg 48
Laundry detergent #2 pg 49
Laundry rinse aid pg 50
Lavender body polish pg 18
Lavender linen water pg 40
Linen spray pg 41

Lip scrub pg 22
Milk bath pg 32
Natural deodorant pg 38
Natural disinfecting spray pg 46
Natural floor cleaning solution pg 58
Natural weed killer pg 60
Oat honey facial mask pg 11
Oatmeal and clay facial scrub pg 17
Peppermint and tea tree foot soak pg 69
Peppermint foot balm pg 34
Positivity Aromatherapy mist pg 80
Purifying aromatherapy air freshener pg 85
Re-hydration drink pg 71
Rose infused witch hazel pg 6
Rose water pg 7
Shampoo bar pg 29
Shea butter and coconut oil hair conditioner pg 24
Sleep aromatherapy roll on pg 83
Spider and critter spray pg 43
Summer body scrub pg 21
Tea mixes pg 76
Toilet cleaner tablets pg 53
Toothpaste #1 pg 25
Toothpaste #2 26
Vapor rub pg 64
Window and glass cleaner pg 57
Wood cutting board cleaner pg 59
Wood polishing spray pg 54
Yogurt mint cucumber facial mask pg 12